By Christopher Dow

Fiction
Effigy
    Book I: Stroud
    Book II: Oakdale
The Books of Bob
    Devil of a Time
    Jumping Jehovah
The Clay Guthrie Mysteries
    The Dead Detective
    Landscape with Beast
    The Texas Troll Unlimited
Roadkill
The Werewolf and Tide, and other Compulsions

Nonfiction
Lord of the Loincloth (nonfiction novel)
Book of Curiosities: Adventures in the Paranormal
Occasional Pilgrimage: Essays on Film, Literature, and Other Matters
Living the Story: The Meandering, True, and Sometimes Strange
    Adventures of an Unknown Writer
    Vol.I: Growing Up Takes a Long Time
    Vol. II: Growing Old Takes Longer

Martial Arts
The Wellspring: An Inquiry into the Nature of Chi
Circling the Square: Observations on the Dynamics of Tai Chi Chuan
Elements of Power: Essays on the Art and Practice of Tai Chi Chuan
Alchemy of Breath: An Introduction to Chi Kung
Leaves on the Wind: A Survey of Martial Arts Literature (Vols. I–VII)

Poetry
City of Dreams
The Trip Out
Texas White Line Fever
Networks
A Dilapidation of Machinery
Puzzle Pieces: Selected Poems

Editor
The Abby Stone: The Poetry of Bartholo Dias
The Best of Phosphene
The Best of Dialog

LEAVES ON THE WIND

volume V

LEAVES ON THE WIND

A Survey of Martial Arts Literature

Volume V

Overviews on Taijiquan
The Taiji Classics

CHRISTOPHER DOW

Phosphene Publishing Company
Temple, Texas

Leaves on the Wind: A Survey of Martial Arts Literature, Volume V

© 2022 by Christopher Dow
ISBN: 978-1-7369307-5-5

All rights reserved. This work may not be copied or otherwise produced or reproduced, in whole or in part, in any form, printed or electronic, without express permission from the publisher, except for brief excerpts used in reviews, articles, and critical works.

Published by:
Phosphene Publishing Company
Temple, Texas, USA
phosphenepublishing.com

1.1

LEAVES ON THE WIND

volume V

Contents

Part I: Overviews of Taijiquan

    The Tao of Tai-Chi Chuan: Way of Rejuvenation——15
        Jou Tsung-hwa

    Fundamentals of Tai Chi Ch'uan——23
        Wen-shan Huang

    Tai Chi Classics——29
        Waysun Liao

    Tai Chi Chuan's Internal Secrets——33
        Doc Fai Wong and Jane Hallander

    Movements of Magic: The Spirit of T'ai-Chi-Ch'uan——37
        Bob Klein

    Heal Yourself and the World with Tai-chi: How to Make Your Life Powerful and Become a Healer——41
        Bob Klein

    The Complete Book of Tai Chi Chuan: A Comprehensive Guide to the Principles and Practice——47
        Wong Kiew Kit

    The Big Book of Tai Chi: Build Health Fast in Slow Motion——55
        Bruce Frantzis

    Genuine Explanations for Authentic Tai Chi——61
        Wu Zhiqing

    The YMCA Taiji Boxing Club's Anniversary Book——69
        The Shanghai YMCA Taiji Boxing Club

    Simple Introduction to Taiji Boxing——71
        Xu Zhiyi

Embrace Tiger, Return to Mountain: The Essence of T'ai Chi——75
  Al Chung-liang Huang

Tai Chi Ch'uan: The Technique of Power——85
  Tem Horwitz & Susan Kimmelman, with H. H. Lui

Methods of Applying Taiji Boxing——89
  Yang Chengfu

T'ai Chi Ch'uan Ta Wen: Questions and Answers on T'ai Chi Ch'uan——93
Answering Questions about Taiji, Including Single Posture Practice Methods
  Chen Weiming

Cheng Tzu's Thirteen Treatises on T'ai Chi Ch'uan——103
Master Cheng's Thirteen Chapters on T'ai-Chi Ch'üan
  Cheng Man-ch'ing

The Tai Chi Book: Refining and Enjoying a Lifetime of Practice——111
  Robert Chuckrow

Tai Chi Dynamics: Principles of Natural Movement, Health, and Self-Development——117
  Robert Chuckrow

Taiji Boxing Explained——123
  Yao Fuchun and Jiang Rongqiao

Essential Concepts of Tai Chi: It is - It is Not - IT IS——127
  William Ting

My Experience of Practicing Taiji Boxing——131
On Studying Taiji's Pushing Hands
  Xiang Kairan

A Study of Taiji Boxing——151
  Long Zixiang

Tai Chi Peng: Root Power Rising——157
  Scott Meredith

The Internal Structure of Cloud Hands: A Gateway to Advanced T'ai Chi Practice——165
  Robert Tangora

Part II: The Taiji Classics

- Biography of Wang Zhengnan (Also known in abridged form as *Boxing Methods of the Internal School*)——171
  Huang Baijia
- Wang Zongyue's Taiji Boxing Treatise: Appended with My Preface and "Five-Word Formula"——173
  Li Yiyu
- The Essence of T'ai Chi Ch'uan: The Literary Tradition——175
  Benjamin Pang Jeng Lo, with Martin Inn, Robert Amacker, and Susan Foe
- T'ai-chi Touchstones: Yang Family Secret Transmissions——177
  Douglas Wile
- Lost T'ai-chi Classics from the Late Ch'ing Dynasty——179
  Douglas Wile
- Taijiquan Theory of Dr. Yang, Jwing-Ming: The Root of Taijiquan——181
  Yang, Jwing-Ming
- Tai Chi Chuan: Decoding the Classics for the Modern Martial Artist——185
  Dan Docherty

PART I

Overviews of Taijiquan

The Tao of Tai-Chi Chuan
Way of Rejuvenation

by Jou Tsung Hwa
(Charles E. Tuttle Co., 1980, 260m pages)

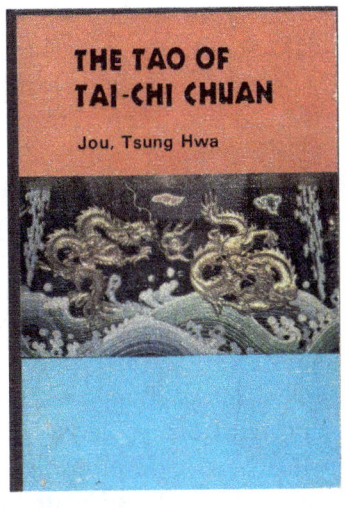

I began practicing Taiji in 1980, the same year that Jou Tsung Hwa published *The Tao of Tai-Chi Chuan*. Thank goodness for that book! Although some aspects of it confused me back then, I thought it was easily the best book in my nascent Taiji library. Since then, my opinion of it has changed slightly, and I now consider it to be one of the three first true classics of Taiji literature in English. The other two are Waysun Liao's *Taichi Classics*, first published in 1977, and Wenshan Huang's *Fundamentals of Tai Chi Ch'uan*, published in 1979. (Both are reviewed below.) If you never bought another book on Taiji beyond these three, you'd be doing just fine.

The Tao of Tai-Chi Chuan opens with Jou's personal journey along the Taiji path. Like so many martial artists, he began to practice to alleviate symptoms of ill health. He subsequently learned Yang Style, then Wu/Hao Style, then the first routine of Chen Style, though he states that he did not practice the latter style to the same extent as Yang and Wu/Hao, which he refers to simply as Wu.

Jou came to the United States in 1972 and began teaching Taiji at Rutgers University, which lasted until 1975. The program ended because the university's curriculum committee, upon reviewing the

Taiji literature then available in English concluded that Taiji was simply a physical exercise and not an area of study worth academic credit. Given the physical focus of the then-current literature, Jou had to concur, but rather than lying down and rolling over, he decided to do something about it. *The Tao of Tai-Chi Chuan* is the result. In the book, Jou aptly demonstrates that Taiji is both exercise and philosophy, and a great deal more.

Chapter one, titled, "Roots," delivers well on its premise of exploring the founding figures of Taiji, beginning, of course, with Chang San-feng. Unlike many writers on Taiji, Jou seems to give more credence to Chang's historicity, but he also acknowledges that a great deal of what has been handed down about Chang is as much legend as it is fact. Even so, his rendition of Chang's life and contributions to internal martial arts is thorough, well-presented, and entertaining.

After discussing Chang, Jou dips farther into the past to explore the roots of internal martial arts prior to Chang. He begins this with Hsa Suanming, a hermit who lived in the Tang Dynasty (618–905) and who developed a thirty-seven movement style called San Hsi Chi that was reportedly similar to Chen Style in its movements. Apparently this was a single posture practice in which the various postures were eventually put together into a sequence.

Other luminaries of proto-internal martial arts who Jou covers are Li Taotze, also of the Tang Dynasty, who created a long chuan called Hsien-Tien Chuan, or, the "Stage Before the Universe Was Created Boxing." Not to be outdone, a later internal style exponent, Hu Chintze, developed Hu-Tien Fa, which means the "Stage After the Universe Was Created Boxing."

After this, Jou jumps to the Chen family, beginning with Chen Wangting, born in the late sixteenth century. His Taiji consisted, Jou says, of five routines. Jou then traces the Chen family through the generations as they further developed and refined their style of internal boxing and narrowed the number of routines to two. He then discusses some of the characteristics of the first routine, from which the others were derived. This is followed by several pages containing small drawings of the first Chen sequence, and this is followed in turn by drawings of the second and much shorter sequence. The drawings are small but well done and have arrows showing the direction of movement of the limbs.

A discussion of the history and characteristics of Yang Style comes next. This begins, of course, with Yang Luchan, and his story will be familiar to anyone who has read much at all on Taiji. But Jou's rendition is fairly detailed and contains several anecdotal stories about Yang's martial encounters, all of which are entertaining. But the harshness of Yang's training of his two surviving sons, Yang Yu and Yang Chian also is highlighted, as are the achievements of his grandsons, particularly Yang Chengfu. If I have a criticism of any of this material, it's that Taiji luminaries of the time sometimes were known by more than one name, and Jou often uses a more obscure version. For example, today Yang Yu is better knows as Yang Panhao, and Yang Chian as Yang Jianhao. The difference in naming conventions can be confusing to those only familiar with the usage that is more common today. The section ends with small but clear drawings of Yang Chengfu performing the long Yang form, also with arrows to indicate the direction the limbs move.

Wu/Hao Style gets the next chapter, and back when I first read this book, I was very confused by it since, at the time, Taiji history was an ocean into which I'd barely inserted a big toe, and it was largely unknown to me. I was then learning what I was told was Wu Style, but it was utterly different from the drawings in Jou's book. Also, although the names in the form list had a familiar ring, they were not in the same sequence as what I was learning.

Over the years, as I studied more about Taiji history, I understood that the Wu Style discussed in Jou's book is what is more commonly known as Wu/Hao or, simply, Hao Style, as opposed to Wu Family Style, which was what I was learning. Although Wu/Hao Style now is more obscure than Yang Style—and even than Wu Family Style—it has a significant place in Taiji history. Both it and Yang Style are the only direct offshoots of Chen Style. Of the other two major Taiji styles, Wu Family Style was developed out of Yang Style, while Sun Style has a complex history that blends Wu/Hao with Bagua and Xingyi. Jou, however, relegates Wu Family and Sun Styles to being mere offshoots rather than individual Taiji styles with unique characteristics that set them apart from their progenitors. As with the Chen and Yang Style sections, this one concludes with a set of small, clear drawings delineating the form.

Jou's intent with the sets of drawings of the various forms is not to instruct in performing a form, but to distinguish visually between the styles. But he does devote the final section of the chapter to the methodology of learning how to perform a Taiji sequence, no matter what style is being practiced. This is worthwhile for anyone taking up Taiji because, as Taiji practitioners know, the form looks easy to do, but it is not. Nor is it easy to learn. It requires devoted and interested practice to learn and become ingrained, and Jou's tips can assist the student in understanding both the short-term and long-term requirements.

Chapter two discusses Taiji philosophy, beginning with the taijitu—the tai chi symbol—and its components: yin and yang. Jou does not stint here, just as he does not stint anywhere in this book. I admit that I'm partial to the beauty and depth of expression that can be discovered in the taijitu, and Jou's examination does not disappoint in either depth or breadth. Included are a number of clear parallels between the taijitu and the art named after it.

The Five Element Theory occupies the next section, and again Jou clearly defines the linkages between the elements themselves and between the elements and a wide variety of philosophical aspects, such as color, season, anatomy, position, and so forth. Next comes a look at the Eight Trigrams, from their history and connection to the *I Ching* to the ways they can be used separately and in combination to help define tangible reality. Jou then goes into the *I Ching*, presenting a basic history, how the text is accessed via the Eight Trigrams, and how the art of Taiji embodies the philosophy expounded by this ancient and revelatory book.

The next section, "The Philosophy of Tai-Chi Chuan," expends the remainder of the chapter on philosophical matters that relate more directly to Taiji. Jou begins the discussion, appropriately enough, by explaining wu-chi, the state of relaxed non-movement in which all movement is possible. He then shows how movement from this quiescent state produces two types of force—yin, or negative force, and yang, or positive force—and how the two forces can interact in different combinations, configurations, and manners to create momentum. Jou then moves on to the Taiji idea of circling the square, or, of "finding the straight in the curved and the curved in the straight." This segues into a look at structural stability and how it can transcend dimensional awareness.

Chapter three is titled, "Foundation." In it, Jou covers a great deal of information critical to the proper practice and functioning of Taiji, beginning with descriptions of eight different types of breathing, each with its own characteristics and effects. They are: Natural Breathing, Cleansing Breathing, Tonic Breathing, Alternate Breathing, Natural Deep Breathing, Long Breathing, Pre-birth or Pre-natal Breathing, and Tortoise Breathing. All are variations of abdominal breathing, but they activate, propel, and process the breath and chi in different ways.

The next section enumerates a number of other Taiji basics, such as naturalness, relaxation, combining the will and chi, establishing solidity in the lower body, slow movement, diligent and regular practice, and moderation in movement. Each is treated to an explanation. This is followed by a thirteen-posture chi kung that utilizes the breathing exercise known as "Heng and Hah." Taiji meditation is covered next, and Jou touches on the elements of the Microcosmic Orbit before moving on to the very useful Chan-ssu Chin, or Reeling Silk Exercise, which he dissects in detail.

From here, Jou segues into the several ways that the practice of Taiji facilitates mental powers and, ultimately, spiritual energy. Linked to this is physical stability, whether one is at rest or is moving. This stability includes stances and how one treats the body in motion as if it is a ball rolling along, constantly maintaining a one-pointed contact with the gravitational pull of the Earth, the tantien serving as the ball's central point. Developing a sense that one is suspended from above allows a more free rotation around one's central equilibrium, and it also allows one to move more rapidly from side to side.

Jou closes out the chapter with a section titled, "The Thirteen Torso Methods," which are additional basic Taiji rules: hollowing the chest, lifting the back, being aware of the crotch region, sheltering the stomach, lifting up the head, skipping, blitzkrieg, relaxing the shoulders, sinking the elbows, positioning the coccyx, and sinking the chi to the tantien. Each is explained in its own paragraph.

A chapter on the Taiji Classics follows. In this, Jou is selective rather than comprehensive, beginning with a classic attributed to Chang San-feng. One by Wang Tsung-yueh, one by Wu Yu-hsing, two by Li Yi-hu, and one by an unknown author follow. Except for the last, Jou provides excellent and often lengthy explanations for the many points presented in these Classics.

"Experiences" is the next chapter, and it contains two sections, each devoted to in-depth Taiji ideas of two significant masters. First is Cheng Man-ch'ing, who conceptualized the development of a Taijiquanist in three stages, each with subsets of advancement. Jou goes into a great deal of detail regarding these, but here I'll simply enumerate them:

I. Human Stage
   1. Lightness
   2. Slowness
   3. Circularity
   4. Constant speed
II. Earth Stage
   1. Agility
   2. Relaxation
   3. The Three Powers
      a. Sinking the weight
      b. Sending the spirit to the crown of the head
      c. Placing the concentration in the tantien
   4. Changes
III. Sky Stage
   1. Sensing emptiness and solidity
   2. Breathing
   3. Consciousness
   4. Void and stillness

The second master that Jou references is Chen Yenlin, and this section is an excerpt from Chen's book, *Tai-Chi Chuan*. This section is ten pages long and covers much of the same basics that Jou and Cheng have already covered, but from a different and illuminating perspective. (Note that Chen Yenlin is also known as Chen Yanlin, Chen Kung, and Yearning K. Chen, so the book Jou is talking about is the one edited diversely by Paul Brennan and Stuart Alve Olson, all reviewed in Volume VI of this series.)

Push Hands is the subject of the final chapter, but the chapter begins with more important basic information regarding the Eight Gates—the eight principal Taiji movement categories—which Jou has touched on previously but here delineates more fully. This was probably the most complete explanation on the Eight Gates in

English-language Taiji literature at the time, and it's still more complete than can be found in almost any Taiji book in English. If I have a problem with any of this material, it's that it describes the Eight Gates in terms of function, which is the standard view of the ways or modes that Taiji manifests chi energy. I prefer to think of the Eight Gates, on the other hand, in terms of dynamics: Where does the energy originate, and where does it end up? But you'll have to read my *Circling the Square: Observations on the Dynamics of Tai Chi Chuan* to learn more about what I mean by that.

After the explanations of the Eight Gates, Jou winds up the book somewhat anticlimactically with push hands itself and how it is done. His explanation is only adequate, but he seems to be simply presenting basic information about push hands rather than trying to give point-by-point instructions.

Throughout the book, Jou salts his explanations with anecdotes and extended metaphors to help get his points across. Some of the anecdotes tell of his interactions with acknowledged masters, such as Cheng Man-ch'ing, while others are word-of-mouth Taiji tales of the great masters. For the most part, the metaphors work well, though a few are, to my mind, somewhat weaker than the others. But weaker or stronger, all illuminate well enough and advance what Jou is talking about. There also are a large number of drawings throughout the book. The form illustrations previously mentioned are well done, but most of the rest of the illustrations tend to be on the crude side. Even so, they are adequate in demonstrating Jou's points. One in particular, showing how energy spirals down through the torso and legs than back up again, was seminal to my understanding of this concept.

In 1983, Jou established the Tai Chi Farm in Warwick, New York , where classes and workshops engaged Taijiquanists from all over the world in many of the deeper aspect of the art. Jou also is the author of *The Tao of Meditation* (reviewed in Volume II of this series) and *The Tao of I Ching*. Jou died in 1998, and two years later, the Tai Chi Farm was sold. But in 2001, his family, students, and friends established the Master Jou Tsung Hwa Memorial Tai Chi Park in Wantage, New Jersey, just twelve miles from the site of the original Tai Chi Farm.

Fundamentals of Tai Chi Ch'uan

by Wen-shan Huang
(South Sky Book Company, 1979, 634 pages)

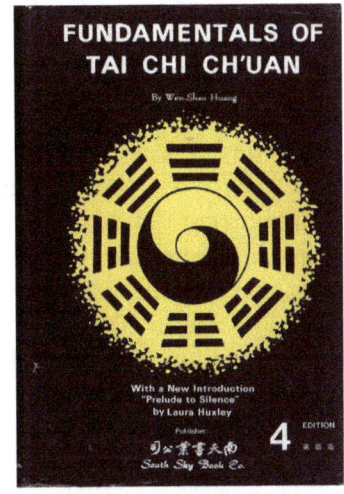

Just as there are giants of Taiji—masters with extraordinarily superb skills—there are giants within Taiji literature. Wen-shan Huang's *Fundamental of Tai Chi Ch'uan* is one of those, standing head and shoulders above most of the others. Even today, almost forty years after the book's first publication, there are few Taiji books that cover the art so thoroughly as Huang's treatise. Or perhaps I ought to call it a tome since, in addition to looming large in importance, it clocks in at a hefty 634 pages.

In addition to being a Taiji exponent, Huang was a sociologist, a cultural theorist, a philosopher, and a legal expert. Before coming to the United States in 1959, he served as dean of the law school at National Sun Yat-sen University and president of Chien Shek University and of the Provincial College of Law and Commerce of Kwangtung. In the U.S., he served on the faculties of the New School in New York and the University of Southern California. He also was the founder and president of the American Academy of Chinese Culture and served as president of the National Tai Chi Ch'uan Association in Los Angeles. The above list of citations only covers about one-third list of the high-level positions he held in academia.

Upon joining the faculty of the University of Southern California in 1959, and in addition to his academic duties, Huang began teaching

Taiji. This marks him as one of the first Taiji instructors in the country. Huang's principal Taiji teacher was Tung Ying Chieh, who was a pupil of Yang Chengfu. However, Huang's introduction lists no fewer than seventeen masters by name "for having imparted their knowledge to me with great generosity." Among the better-known of these in America are Cheng Man-ching, Da Liu, and T. T. Liang. Clearly, Huang's understanding of Taiji is deep, and his academic background is apparent in his erudite and thorough writing style.

The book opens with eight (!) essays variously labeled as introductions, prefaces, notes, acknowledgements, and author biography. The first is by Laura Huxley (Mrs. Aldous Huxley), several are by academic associates of Huang, and two are by Huang himself. The author bio is uncredited. Most of this prefatory material is simply laudatory of Huang, but in his own introductions, the author lays out the basic principles of Taiji and his purposes in writing the book.

The book is broken into four parts followed by a thick section of appendices. "Part I: Historical and Philosophical," begins with a chapter that defines Taiji as an art of life and then goes on to discuss in elementary terms the idea of form or structure, the techniques of bodily movement, breathing, self-defense, and the therapeutic value of Taiji. The material here is somewhat cursory, but it is intended to introduce the reader to basic concepts rather than to fully discuss them. He leaves the more intense examinations of the art for subsequent chapters.

Those begin with one of the most thorough historical surveys of Taiji that exists outside of books completely devoted to the subject. In it, Huang delineates the origins of the Chinese martial arts in general before discussing the differences between the "exoteric" and "esoteric" schools of martial arts. After that, he gets down to brass tacks on the development of Taiji itself. This stuff is clearly written by someone with access to old Chinese documents on the development of Taiji, and Huang's presentation of the material is thorough.

The next chapter discusses Taiji's relationship to the *I Ching*. After setting the stage with several pages of introductory remarks, Huang delves into the history of the *I Ching* and the combination of cosmic law and ethical considerations inherent in that ancient text. From there, he moves on to Taiji's relationship to the tai chi symbol.

Huang favors the more elaborate tai chi diagram created by Chou Tun-yi rather than the more familiar taijitu depicting two fish shapes rotating within a circle. The latter, he states, "has no practical value, except that it represents Yin and Yang." Chou's diagram, on the other hand, "embraces all the abstruse principles" of Taiji. I tend to disagree, but this isn't the place to digress on that subject. (For those who are interested in a discourse on the two-fish taijitu, check out my essay, "Symbolic Movement" in *Elements of Power: Essays on the Art and Practice of Tai Chi Chuan*.)

Huang then goes into the basic principles of Taiji in relation to Confucianism, Taoism, and Zen Buddhism. This is fascinating material that is too complex to easily or succinctly paraphrase, so I won't attempt to do so, but it includes in-depth discussions of the principles of breath control, serenity and emptiness, softness, and non-striving and non-aggression, among others. Taiji's effects on health follow, and here Huang looks at the art's impact on the central nervous system, the circulatory and respiratory systems, digestion, and metabolism. The next chapter examines Taiji in light of modern philosophy and science, including the physical, biological, psychological, and ethical aspects of Taiji.

Part II is titled "Methodological and Theoretical," and here the author looks closely at several issues: "The Method of the Torso," "The Method of the Fist," "The Method of the Palms," "The Method of the Legs," "The Method of the Feet," and "The Method of the Steps." Each part succinctly dissects its subject and contains very valuable information. Taiji's general operational methodology follows. I'll simply list his subject matter in this section:

1. In postures, the trunk is upright, erect, comfortable. Body and mind are relaxed and calm.
2. All actions should be light, nimble, and alert, emphasizing continuity, flexibility, circling, and unity.
3. Actions are adjusted to breathing and the unity of the internal and the external.
4. The breath is deep and natural—the chi is directed by the mind to sink downward to the tantien.
5. Cultivating the chi, harmonizing the breath, and the controlling of the mind and spirit inwardly are crucial.
6. The chi is excited in its circulation in the body.
7. In practicing the exercise, the spirit should be absolutely integrated and the hands and eyes should be coordinated.

8. The waist/spine structure is the chief controller of bodily movements.
9. The method of stepping mainly emphasizes lightness, nimbleness, circling, and stability.
10. The art facilitates interaction of the conjugate powers of yin and yang, the harmonizing of the dynamic and static with the direction of the mind, and the complimentary nature of yielding (pliability) and unyielding (hardness).
11. The Thirteen Postures.
12. The operations of Wardoff, Rollback, Press, and Push.
13. The operations of the Pull, Split, Elbow Stroke, and Shoulder Stroke.
14. The circular movements of "Reeling of Silk" exercises.
15. In the joint hands operations (push hands), attention has to be paid to the techniques known as "to adhere and lift," "to join," "to adhere horizontally," "to attach from the rear," and "neither let go nor resist."
16. The stages of comprehension and application of the intrinsic energies.

The list itself is informative enough on the surface, but each of these subjects is treated in depth over the course of one to several pages, opening their topics like flowers unfolding to reveal their essences. Breathing is the topic of the next two chapters, and as with the previous chapter, the text delves the greater depths of the subject.

The form instruction section occupies the next chapter, and it depicts a long Yang form and includes detailed text accompanied by excellent photographs. Right in the middle of this section is a foldout sheet that shows the foot-stepping pattern for the entire form. These sorts of charts often seem to me to be superfluous at best, and practically worthless at worst, and this one is no different.

A longish chapter displaying possible applications for many of the movements comes next, and it is rather more complete than is usual for this kind of material. The applications are followed by a chapter on push hands that shows two-handed push hands, four corners (Tui Shou), Ta Lu, and free-style. As with the applications section, this is fairly detailed, and inexperienced practitioners without an instructor to teach these aspect of Taiji might actually be able to study this material and learn how to push hands.

Self-defense is the subject of the final chapter. This chapter is a "tell" rather than a "show," and it discusses the main characteristics of Taiji pugilism, strategy, non-opposition, non-separation, circular movement, Central Equilibrium, speed, intrinsic energy, and what Huang terms the "Three Stages of Applying Energy," which are feinting, neutralizing, and borrowing energies.

So far, we've worked our way up to page 425, and the more than 200 pages that remain are taken up by various appendices. The first three are the first three of the Taiji Classics in very thorough translations. Huang then delivers an essay on the Classics, discussing their history, enumerating them, and finally translating one more for the reader.

The chapter that follows is, essentially, it's own little book titled *The Art of Glowing Health*. In it, Huang presents a modern system of balanced exercise, self-massage, and breathing rhythms drawn from the wisdom of Taoism, Zen, and acupuncture. Comprising forty-four pages of text with numerous illustrations, it discusses internal exercise in general and then gives instruction in the Ten Fundamental Treasures (a chi kung series) and several other exercises, some of which also are found in the well-known Eight Pieces of Brocade chi kung form. The chapter ends with self-massage techniques.

"Cultural Breathing" is the title of the next chapter, and it discusses at length the subjects of abdominal breathing, chi circulation through both the Microcosmic and Macrocosmic Orbits, and the effects and benefits of abdominal breathing on the body's various internal systems. The concept of longevity takes up the following chapter, and here Huang lays out a great deal of scientific research done up to that time on the subject of gerontology. Much of this latter material may be dated now.

The development of condensed or abbreviated Taiji forms finds a few pages here before Huang gives space to his final subjects, which are covered here by other authors: the effects of isometric exercise on hypertension, circulation, and claudication, which refers to the impairment in walking, or pain, discomfort, numbness or tiredness in the legs caused by poor circulation. This material is rather technical but is worth perusing.

Fundamentals of Tai Chi Ch'uan is a wonderful book and an important one, but it isn't a perfect book. Its exegesis of the art of Taiji is thorough and deep, but there are technical issues with the production. It was produced in the days before computerized typesetting, and there are a great number of typographical errors, inconsistencies, and oddities strewn throughout its pages. Further, there are numerous inconsistencies in spelling that are important and should have been caught by better editing. For example, Huang acknowledges his friend Yung-cheng Kwang for posing for the push hands photos, but later in the same paragraph, he refers to him as Mr. Kwong. Which one is it? The book also contains material that seems to be dross for a volume aimed at an English-speaking audience, such as the inclusion of twenty pages of Chinese text followed by a several-page bibliography also in Chinese, that replicates material already presented in English.

But these are relatively minor matters when compared to the significance of the information Huang imparts. Unfortunately, the book seems to be out of print at this time, which is a crying shame. Used copies of the various editions that appeared between 1979 and the mid to late 1980s run from about $60 to $80. That's a lot to spend on a book, but you might want to spend it anyway since Taiji books don't get much more thorough than this one.

Tai Chi Classics

by Waysun Liao
(Golden Oak Productions, 1977, 300 pages)
(Shambhala Classics, 2001, 224 pages)

I began practicing Taiji early in 1980, and as soon as I did, I began acquiring books on the subject. Most at the time were simple beginner's manuals: relatively basic glosses on the history, philosophy, and principles of the art accompanied by a series of photos or drawings depicting the author's Taiji form. Some of these are better than others. Waysun Liao's *Tai Chi Classics* isn't one of those better ones. It's much better. In fact, at the time of its initial publication, it was one of the five best books on Taiji available in English, all of which form, along with the several versions of the Taiji Classics, the founding core of Taiji literature in English. These are the books that showed the rest of us writers the kinds of thoroughness and informational quality we should aspire to.

I recently reread it to see if I still thought that way, only to discover that it's even better. That might be because I understand Taiji more now and can appreciate some of Liao's statements that passed over my head in the early

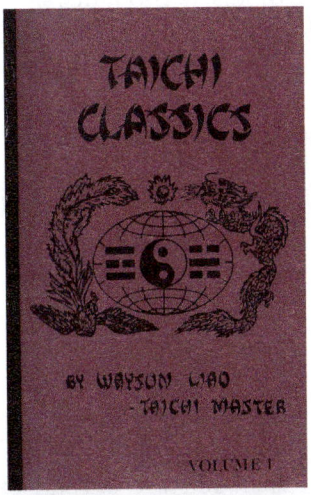

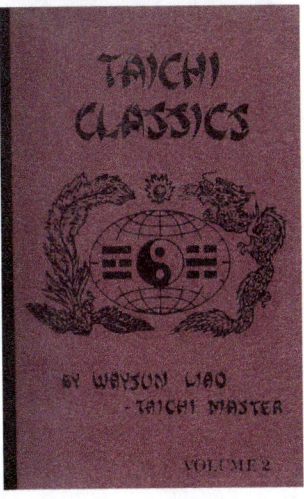

1980s. But that's not to say that the book was abstruse when I first read it. It isn't, and in fact, it provided me several keys to advancement and imparted to me some of my earliest understandings of how Taiji functions on its more subtle levels. I probably ought to say here that the title is a bit misleading in that, while some of the Taiji Classics (the old ones, I mean) are included here, most of the book consists of Liao's thoughts.

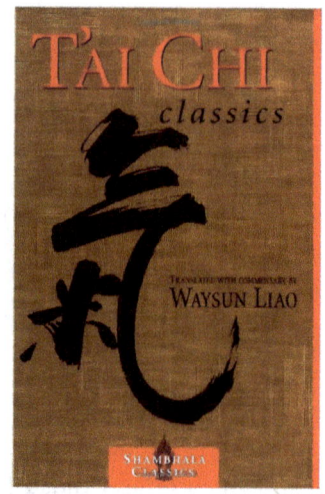

Liao opens the book with a chapter on Taiji's background. It is a fairly thorough discussion of the historical, philosophical, and cultural milieu out of which Taiji arose, but he deemphasizes the role of famous Taiji families (Chen, Yang, Wu, etc.) in furthering and disseminating Taiji in favor of a historical view that places the development of the art in the Wu Tang Mountains—this despite the fact that the form depicted in the second half of the book appears to be a fairly traditional Yang Style.

Next is a chapter on chi, beginning with a definition that includes the concepts of li and jin. He then discusses breathing, which is critical to Taiji, and the idea of the mind leading the chi. Included are several exercises to improve breathing and to condense the chi within the body. He then goes into a section on the internal workings of Taiji, and winds up the chapter with methods to increase chi awareness that include an excellent and detailed exposition of how breathing functions to amplify and propel chi through the body.

He then discusses jin and internal power at length. This was almost unheard of in other Taiji books at the time of original publication, and this chapter is still highly informative. There may be a few more-recent books that go into greater depth or detail on jin than this, but this is still a decent rendition that fairly successfully attempts to apply the principles of physics to Taiji—again, a relatively new concept in Taiji books of the day.

This chapter is followed by a long and solid translation of key Taiji Classics (the old ones, I mean) accompanied by commentary from the author on the meanings and concepts of these old documents. Again, this level of interpretation was generally not available in other Taiji books of the time, which has kept the book relevant despite its age. After all, Taiji is timeless, so a good book on it is timeless, too.

Finally, the book ends with the requisite series of illustrations of the form—in this case, crude line drawings rather than photos—and descriptive text. Despite the simplicity of the illustrations, they are done well enough and include arrows to indicate the direction of movement. The descriptive text is good, and the whole series is fairly detailed should you care to notice. But even if you completely ignore this section, which I pretty much did since I don't practice Yang Style, the rest of the book is so good that skipping this chapter doesn't make the book seem slighter.

This review is based on the first edition of *Tai Chi Classics*, which was, essentially, a self-published effort. This was in those prehistoric days before personal computers, much less the Internet and on-demand publishing, and the book exhibits primitive production values in contrast to the excellence of the material. The type was set on a typewriter, with typographical errors simply struck over rather than erased and replaced, and the illustrations are all crude line drawings by the author. But as simple as they are, the drawings manage to convey Liao's points. The book was printed in two volumes via photocopier, each volume bound with plastic strips. I'm not sure why Liao didn't find a real publisher for this book at the time because it was a lot better than 95 percent of the other books out there. And still is.

Apparently, though, he finally did find a publisher: none other than Shambhala Books, which republished it in 2001. (The cover of that edition is shown above.) The fact that a publisher of this caliber has reissued the work speaks to its excellence. I do not currently have a copy of the reissue so I can't do a real comparison between the two editions, but I did glance through the few pages I could see on the Amazon site. It seems that it's pretty much the same book but with a few improvements—namely the typesetting—which can't be bad when you start out with something this good. I didn't see any of the drawings in the pages I could look at, so I don't know if they're the same as in the original edition or if they have been updated, too, with better drawings or photographs. No matter. It's still a great Taiji book.

Tai Chi Chuan's Internal Secrets

by Doc Fai Wong and Jane Hallander
(Unique Publications, 1991, 124 pages)

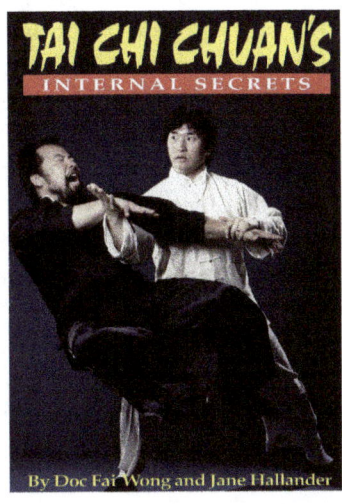

At this stage of my reading on Taiji, I tend to go for books that are heavy on history, philosophy, and dynamics. The title of *Tai Chi Chuan's Internal Secrets* was intriguing, and its authors are both expert and well respected. I'd read a lot of their columns and articles in American martial arts magazines back in the 1980s and 1990s, and I thought they frequently delivered some good information despite the limited scope possible in a magazine article. Certainly, Wong has an impressive background, and Hallander not much less. But I have to say that, for a couple of reasons, this book did not meet my expectations.

The first reason concerns the authors' idiosyncratic take on Taiji history, which is the subject of the first chapter. Taiji history can be a sticky subject with some practitioners, mostly because the actual history of Taiji prior to the mid 17th century is not clearly delineated by actual historical documentation—or at least none that is publicly known. Hence, a great deal of Taiji "history" is a farrago of supposition, inference, legend, and wishful thinking.

Here is not the place to go into an exposition on the history of Taiji, but it is the place to note that the extensive and far-flung history given in this book matches almost no other history I've read. If you think Chang San-feng was a problematic historical figure as the creator of Taiji, then you might be predisposed to take with a hefty grain of salt a specifically detailed Taiji history that goes as much as 800 years farther into the past. Further, this history cites people and writings that seemed to have escaped the notice of professional historians on the subject of Taiji history. Once the history gets to the Chen family, though, it settles into a fairly routine recitation of the development of Taiji by the founders of several of the major styles.

Okay. I'm not enough of a scholar of Taiji history to debate the specific historical points in this chapter, but I tend to like to see a little corroboration from alternate sources, and I might be hard-pressed to do that in this case. Maybe Wong and Hallander have access to historical documents that others aren't aware of or privy to. If so, they should share them with the Taiji community at large in an effort to clear up some of the obfuscation surrounding the art's insemination, development, and dissemination.

Chapter two is titled: "Taiji's Internal Secrets," but I have to say that the "secrets" in this book aren't really secrets but simply basic principles and rules for correct form practice. Many are tenets from the Taiji Classics restated in more straightforward language. In this respect, the book was probably fairly informative at the time of its first publication. But these days, these principles and rules can be found—equally well or better stated—in scores of books on Taiji and chi kung, and in the dozens of versions of the Taiji Classics available in English. The chapter opens with a recitation of the way students learned Taiji in the past and relates that Yang Chenfu altered this learning process, all of which would be more interesting if it actually led to some Taiji "secrets" instead of forming the bulk of the chapter, which then finishes with several paragraphs describing the difference between Taiji and chi kung.

The next two chapters, however, work hard to save the book. Chapter three details three meditational postures that might be termed "still chi kungs" and four breathing exercises that might be termed "moving chi kungs." Chapter four shows ten martial stances designed to increase balance, chi flow, leg strength, and stamina. At my age, I pretty much stick with some warmups, the Taiji form, and the several chi kungs that I do, but I settled on these after working and experimenting with a lot of others over the years. I've always thought that changing up one's routine is nothing but beneficial.

The exercises in this chapter are the kinds that will improve your Taiji movements and assist in ramping up your chi flow. When Wong and Hallander present practical material, their expertise shines, and they present this material well enough that one could learn to do these helpful exercises from their descriptions.

Unfortunately, the authors then waste fifty-four pages—about 45 percent of the book—with a photo series of Wong performing a long Yang Style. Wong was expert then (and undoubtedly is even more expert now), so the postures are pretty impressive. If one cares to look. It seems that until 2000, such a series of photos was obligatory, since nearly every book on Taiji that appeared before then had one. I can understand including a series to aid the author's students in learning a particular style, but this series isn't really detailed enough to be a good learning tool.

And even depicting specific postures for other purposes—such as comparison—is problematic. Wong is expert, and so are others, and there can be many discrepancies in the outward appearance of any given movement—even between two Taiji players performing the same form. As experienced Taiji players know, the postures are just outward expressions of internal energy. Sure, we need to learn how to perform the form accurately, but just what is "accurate?" Wong's postures don't look exactly like Yang Chenfu's, for example, but does that make them wrong? Very likely, both are right. Style specifics, body type, and intent all come into play in a given posture, making such series of photos moot for anyone not practicing exactly the same style, or one that is very similar.

It could be argued that it is informative to study the postural differences between styles or between different versions of the same style, but I think that photos are not an adequate means of delivering such information. Film and video are much more effective in showing dynamic movement, which is the real key, not the static final or intermediate postures. So I can't help but fault this book for the inclusion of the series of form photos. There isn't even the pretense of a secret here, and in the end, this chapter just seems like filler to expand a very slender volume that might otherwise have looked like a few articles from *Inside Kung Fu* bound together under one cover. Even the cover photo reinforces this impression.

Chapter six, "Correct Form Practice," however, brings back some real information. Still no secrets, but the information is solid and useful, at least for beginners. It primarily concerns correcting faulty body alignments—especially those that affect the body's foundation and ability to root—then moves on to how relaxation enhances chi flow and how intent helps direct the chi properly. This information is good, but again it's also pretty basic.

Chapters seven and eight discuss applications and push hands respectively, using both words and photos. As with photos of form postures, photos of applications and push hands are practically worthless as learning aids unless you already have enough experience with Taiji that the techniques are already familiar. And in that case, you don't need the photos. Anybody who has pushed hands very much or done any sparring knows that nothing works quit right, anyway, when you're in motion with another person. You have to feel the action and reaction. Martial arts movies and various videos of applications and techniques, such as those on *YouTube*, are far more useful for learning how to make the moves work against an opponent than are static pictures. So, as with chapter five, these two chapters seem like filler. But, of course, there was no *YouTube* when this book was published.

All-in-all, this book reflects its age. Anybody who has pursued Taiji for more than a few years will find little that is new or useful here —except, perhaps, the chi kung exercises in chapters three and four. But for beginner and intermediate students, these two chapters and the chapter on correct form practice can provide some useful and fairly well-explicated tools to further their practice. Just be aware that half this slender volume is not going to give you much at all.

And really, there is only one secret to Taiji: Practice.

Movements of Magic
The Spirit of T'ai-Chi-Ch'uan

by Bob Klein
(Newcastle Publishing Co., 1984, 158 pages)

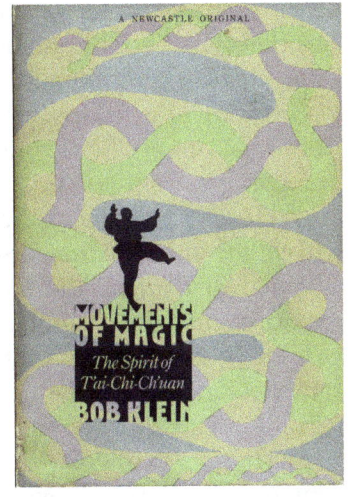

Bob Klein's *Movements of Magic* was one of the earliest philosophical books in English on Taiji. In many respects, it, along with only a handful of other books from the same time period, virtually defined Taiji literature of this sort for the English-speaking audience.

The purpose of this sort of book is not to give basic historical background and delineate form, as is the case with most beginner category of Taiji books. Nor does it deal specifically with technique, martial usage, or specific physical and energy dynamics of the art, as do the nuts-'n-bolts category of books. Obviously, Taiji is a syncretic art, so some elements of these types of books might be present in a a philosophical work, but the real purpose of such books is to relate musings on the subject of Taiji, often from a personal perspective.

Klein was a student, most notably, of William C. C. Chen, who certified him to teach. He opened the Long Island School of Tai-chi-Chuan in 1975, and the school is still operational, making it one of the longest-running Taiji schools in the U.S.—nearly fifty years!

Klein's purpose in *Movements of Magic* is not to talk about the movements, techniques, energy, or martial aspects of Taiji, per se, though he touches on all of these. Instead, he uses the space to discuss

Taiji in relation to personal and cultural beliefs, self-awareness, and personal and spiritual development. He writes in the preface:

> T'ai-chi-Ch'uan is not a belief system or dogma, but a series of techniques designed to tap into and channel the powers of nature, both within and around us.... T'ai-chi-Ch'uan reconnects the mind to the body, the consciousness to the subconscious and the individual to his environment.

Throughout the course of the subsequent six chapters, he attempts to do just that with his interpretation of the art.

In chapter one, titled "The Form (I)," Klein delves into how the Taiji form develops certain qualities in the practitioner, including smoothness of motion, looseness of the body, concentration, rooting, a sense of internal energy, elasticity, breath control, and connectedness. Each aspect is give its own explication, and in the section on rooting, he outlines an exercise designed to develop or increase one's sense of this very important skill.

He also introduces the concept of the Body Mind—as distinct from the mind in the head—that controls, or can be allowed or trained to control, the movements of the body. Considerable advancements have taken place in understanding what the Body Mind is since Klein wrote this book, but he was prescient in implying that it is, essentially, the tantien. We can now understand it as a major neural plexus located in the belly called the Enteric Nervous System. In advocating for the Body Mind, Klein shows how the head mind is like a possessive ruler who refuses to share power, to the detriment of the organism. True power is power shared throughout a body system—particularly with the Body Mind—allowing the entire body system to function optimally.

Tied up in all this is the idea of letting go—letting go of preconceptions, of false protections, of self, of addiction to the mind. As this is accomplished, one begins to open to both the self and to the world in ways that benefit both.

Chapter two—"The Form (II)"—begins with ways to turn the attention of the Body Mind to emotions and memory in an effort to reconnect the self to a more basic reality. Tied up in this is the use of the mind, which can be redirected from its self-centered ruminations to more worthy tasks, such as directing the internal energy that one becomes more aware of once the thinking mind relinquishes control to the Body Mind. This leads to a discussion of centering and, of course, the tantien and the importance of this structure in generating and mobilizing chi energy.

Interestingly, Klein advocates practicing the form in different ways, not just in its standard mode, to broaden the practitioner's understanding. Slanting Form over-emphasizes the back-and-forth seesawing to train balance and counter balance. Old Man Form is done as if one were weak and sick. Snake Form emphasizes a slinky elasticity. Monkey Form emphasizes bending without losing balance. And Closed Eyes Form is done—well, you get the picture even if you can't see it. There are a few more, and all work with one or two primary elements of Taiji to magnify and expand their influence over the practitioner's body, mind, and emotions.

Chapter three is "Push Hands," but there are no photos of partners squaring off. Instead, Klein discusses the lessons of push hands, such a yielding, neutralization, and pushing, all of which open what he calls a "field of sensitivity" to one's opponent. This leads the exponent into the realm of spontaneity. Rooting and the interplay of yin and yang come in, and then Klein presents a few push hands exercises that partners can practice to further refine their skills. Along the way, he also discusses "hiding" from the opponent, tension, and feigning vulnerability.

"Kung Fu" is the next chapter, and in it, Klein talks more about kung fu as self-development. He also presents a dozen kung fu exercises done mostly with partners that help develop fighting skills. After that, he discusses the mechanics of fighting, including several exercises to improve kicking skills. All of this, he says, is to develop instinctual fighting, which, after a time, turns into magical fighting.

Healing is the subject of chapter five. In it, Klein does not disparage Western medicine but shows that harmonizing one's energy with that of others and one's environment can produce the greatest healing effects. There is a lot of psychology in this chapter as well as how cultural and social factors can enhance or inhibit energy flow and health in addition to directing beliefs. Wrapped up in this discussion is the idea that personal helplessness and the need to constantly win are both losing strategies that hold a person back from a greater sense of fulfillment and accomplishment.

The psychological aspect might also seem to be the topic of the book's final chapter, "The Evolution of the Human Mind," but that's not the case. Instead, the chapter talks about the role of the mind in spiritual alchemy and personal development and the effects those have on one's world view. Included is a discussion of the meaning of the "Five Elements" of Chinese philosophy and how they relate to mental and spiritual advancement.

This leads into a comparative discussion of Western and Eastern mysticism that takes in elements as diverse as the purpose and meaning of ritual, the Qabala, the Tarot, astrology, the astral body, and mythology, just to name a few. The goal here is to harmonize these various world views by identifying their very basic similarities.

In some ways, *Movements of Magic* is like an intense self-help book that uses Taiji as the mechanism for that help. In it, Klein covers a lot of ground, but he always seems grounded thanks to his down-to-earth language and the entertaining and illuminating anecdotes that advance the ideas he presents. This is a worthwhile read, even for more experienced practitioners, and its ideas remain valid for me, even decades after first reading it.

Heal Yourself and the World with Tai-chi
How to Make Your Life Powerful and Become a Healer

Bob Klein
(Long Island School of Tai-Chi and Pilates, 2021, 430 pages)

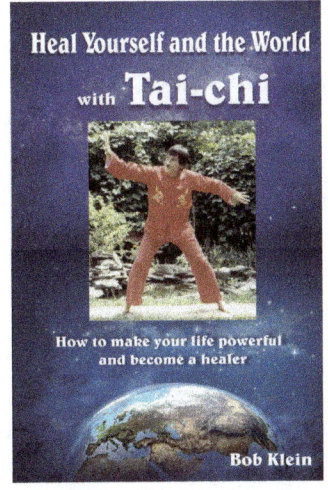

Bob Klein is a longtime Taiji teacher and author living on Long Island, New York. He was part of the first flowering of tai chi in America and was an early contributor to original tai chi literature in English. His first book, *Movements of Magic*, is reviewed above. The following thumbnail bio is from his school's website:

> Bob Klein has been studying healing, meditation, Tai-chi and Kung-fu since the 1960's. He received his Tai-chi-Chuan teaching certificate from Grandmaster William C.C. Chen in 1975. He also studied with healers from several nature-oriented cultures. His career began as a zoologist, studying animal behavior at Cornell University, the New York Zoological Society and the Smithsonian Tropical Research Institute. He would travel to the jungles of Central America to study the wildlife. Mr. Klein was attracted to Tai-chi because it is based on the movements of animals. He is the author of four books on Tai-chi and healing and has produced over 60 instructional videos. Mr. Klein has been featured in such magazines as *Inside Kung-fu*, *Tai-chi Magazine* & *Dao Magazine*.

Klein's bio does not delve into his career as a zoologist, but as the book under consideration shows, his association with animals became a prime motivator of his life and a serious adjunct to his study of Taiji, chi kung, and other traditional methods of healing. Klein has been places that revealed much to him, and he wants you to visit, too.

With most martial arts books, I can tell you what it's about, but I can't with this one. Most martial arts book have a "plot": a preface, history and precepts of the martial art, and a teaching section. That's a book about something. So is a book that discusses specific techniques, kinetics, or other aspect of a martial art. But not this one. This one isn't really about anything. It's more about everything. And while this is a Taiji book, you can't read it to learn about Taiji, though you will definitely pick up some good information and pointers along the way. Instead, this book uses Taiji and Klein's own chi kung system, Zookinesis, to extrapolate about healthy and fulfilling ways to approach and live life. For him, Taiji is a large part of that. So I can't really review *Healing Yourself and the World with Tai-chi* in the conventional sense, merely characterize it.

There is a touch of the memoir in these pages, but the book is not autobiographical—not unless you call it autobiophilosophical. Klein doesn't lay out a narrative of his life, which might be pretty interesting on its own, but many of his life experiences appear in the book. For example, he often refers to different aspect of the several years he spent studying and collecting wild animals in Central America and of his animal-related experiences later in life. He uses these experiences—and many anecdotes and fine metaphors—to amplify or illustrate the ideas and concepts he brings to the fore.

Essentially, Klein writes books that aren't about how to do Taiji, but rather are about what Taiji can do for you and what the art means in the context of a fuller life and a broader sense of reality. In taking this stance, Klein is planted firmly within the Taoist/shamanic tradition, and this book can be considered a distillation of the characteristics of that archetype. You can't approach this book as if you're going to read it, nor is it the sort of book you look in for information, though there is plenty of information at every turn to keep it solid. Instead, it is a series of extended, freeform meditations using Taiji principles that find focus in several areas. This is a book that has to be absorbed.

Is it a Taiji book? Yes. Is it a "self-help"—or rather, let's call it "self-realization"—book? Yes. Is it a philosophical world view? Again, yes. But reader beware: This is not a book to take for a Sunday spin. It's a cross-country journey.

Klein's ideas and concepts unfold over the course of nine long chapters. That number reminds me of the Taiji concept of the Nine-channel Pearl, a metaphor used to indicate the passage of the chi, from foot to fingertips, through the nine major joints of the body: ankle, knee, hip, shoulder, elbow, wrist, and three joints of the phalanges. Each of these chapters is its own meditation as the reader is led, like the chi, to the conclusion of all nine. And what is that conclusion? I think what Klein is getting at on a basic level is to encourage readers to connect with their deeper, truer selves and to live a life that is replete with awareness and vitality. And he wants to give you some tools to help you do just that.

Certainly the book is replete with awareness and vitality. I hadn't read more than twenty pages before Klein's onslaught of positive thinking and vibes began to invade my dark spaces and poke them awake. He covers so many ideas that the prose almost reads like stream-of-consciousness. Sometimes I couldn't read more than a sentence or two without becoming so involved in the ideas that my thoughts constantly took off on some tangent or other. I don't usually talk back to books, but frankly, I didn't read this book so much as have a dialogue with it on many subjects of intense interest to me. Despite my having said that this book isn't one to take out for a Sunday spin, I suspect that you can open it at random, start reading, and find something interesting, important, provocative, or relevant.

Throughout the book, one of Klein's major touchstones is Zookinesis, which is a chi kung system he developed after years of working professionally with animals. From what I gather, Zookinesis is a set of chi kung based on animal movements. In this, it is akin to many kung fu and chi kung styles based on the movements of animals, but there is a major difference. Zookinesis takes into account not just the physicality specific to a particular animal, but also that animal's intrinsic behaviors and the ways its spirit manifests. Its emotions. You'll actually learn something about animal behavior—particularly the behavior of snakes—by reading this book.

There are Taiji lessons here, but not in the conventional sense. There are no chapters on how to do this or that, and there might be a good reason. "Sometimes the principles of Tai-chi can be more challenging to a student than the exercises," Klein writes, and so he concentrates on the principles, though not in a straightforward manner. Just as he drops in ideas gleaned from his interactions with animals, specific Taiji lessons are strewn along the way, with plenty of good tips and suggestions, all well explicated. Using his conversational writing style to advantage, Klein reminds us of a great many Taiji precepts—some macro, some micro, but all important to keep in mind—and he does this by subtly weaving the ideas into whole cloth. Push hands, for example, is the subject of a long section of the first chapter, and the text offers valuable advice on personal dynamics during push hands in a depths that I've never encountered before in a book.

Klein saves most of his more specific Taiji instruction for the final chapter, "Review of Internal Mechanics." But this isn't to say that this chapter is overtly instructional. Instead, it's what might be termed "operational." In other words, it is more about how Taiji creates structural and dynamic opportunities for defeating an enemy, rather than telling you how to do a specific form, movement, or application. Also appearing here and there are various exercises—mostly chi kung forms—to help you open and energize your body, mind, and spirit. There is wisdom here, and even if you know some of this stuff already, it's good to be reminded that life can be made better by understanding that tension and ego are the enemies—not just of Taiji, but of life. And throughout, Klein encourages the reader to adhere to that venerable Taiji phrase: Invest in loss.

Another Taiji precept—stand like a mountain, flow like a great river—can be used to describe Klein's prose. As I said earlier, the writing here is almost stream-of-consciousness, and if he isn't quite the William Faulkner of martial arts literature, his prose is densely written. Or rather, the writing isn't dense in the sense of being complex so much it relates ideas and concepts that are weighty and densely layered. However, the words and phrases he uses to get those ideas and concepts across are easy to digest.

If Klein sometimes seems repetitive or meandering, it's usually because he consistently addresses the same sets of issues from different angles. Occasionally, I thought he could have trimmed the text a bit to make it less repetitive in spots, but the truth is that we all keep returning to touchstones of our lives. A certain amount of repetition is fine, particularly since Klein keeps thing moving and comes back to concepts with insights lent by perspectives that otherwise might not be noticed using a single-angle approach. In almost every instance, the sum of the different approaches infuses the book with clues on how to live a holistic way of life that includes healing and all the other aspect that help make life worthwhile. And just when he seems to be circling around a subject, he suddenly spirals in on its core characteristics and lessons. Finally, regarding the writing, his authorial voice, while straightforward and encouraging, is salted with touches of friendly humor.

Do I believe everything Klein writes? No. After reading some of his statements, I often wished he was present so we could discuss some of the finer points. For example, he talks of achieving a high —and heightened—state of being, but I have to say that oftentimes such heights seem out of reach of all but the super-dedicated and fortunate few. So what about the rest of us whose aim isn't to become masters, but simply to enhance our lives? And I sometimes found myself thinking that he has this or that wrong, or skewed, at least, and often I wanted to say to him, "Yeah, but what about…?" I can be a cynical sort. But then he's off onto something that totally resonates with my experiences in life and with Taiji. He's generally right—or right enough—that my complaints usually just dissipated by the next sentence.

And like I said, I constantly found my mind sparked by what Klein was saying and then wandering off into its own territory. I appreciate any book that makes me think, and the fact that this one did that constantly demonstrates for me the viability of the ideas and concepts he expresses. And the truth is, often my quibbles are of a purely writerly nature. Klein, in the final analysis, has much to say, and he most often says it well, and I'm fully convinced that anyone who tries to get others to look more deeply into themselves and life—not just mere existence—is worth listening to.

Klein states that the book is intended for anyone, not just Taiji folks, who seeks a fuller life. In the end, I'd have to call this book an extended pep talk and sales pitch—not for a product (unless you count Taiji and chi kung as products), but for a relaxed and open mind that isn't locked into self-destructive patterns. The real product is your own well-being. However, it seems to me that much of the Taiji-specific material in the book will go right over the heads of non-Tai-Chi folks, and even Taiji beginners. To my mind, the Tai-Chi-specific material will be more useful to intermediate, and even lower-level advanced students. Certainly books for those levels of students are rare enough.

I'm not endorsing Klein's methods, just this book, which I think is a worthy addition to any martial arts library. In it, Klein gives sage and practical advice for the practice of Taiji and a formula for living more fully, both embedded in an unrelentingly positive message.

Did I learn from this book? Yes. And I was reminded of things I already knew but had stored away and temporarily forgotten. Not only was it good to be reminded, Klein's prose, densely packed with ideas, concepts, and insights, is an excellent vehicle to convey them.

I think Bob Klein's world is highly idealized, though the reality around us obviously is not. But what Klein is really saying is that in life, as in Taiji, we should strive for relaxed and spontaneous perfection and keep lofty goals in mind, in sight, in body, and in practice—not only for the sake of our own well-being and souls, but for the benefit of the world and others. Taiji, he believes, can be a vehicle to help effect that sort of change, transforming a world of ego and aggression into one of peaceful coexistence, in which we all have the opportunity to forge ahead into a more personally and socially productive and rewarding way of life.

I like to think he's right. We sure could use more of that peaceful coexistence in the world right now.

The Complete Book of Tai Chi Chuan
A Comprehensive Guide to the Principles and Practice

By Wong Kiew Kit
(2002, Tuttlle Publishing, 318 pages)

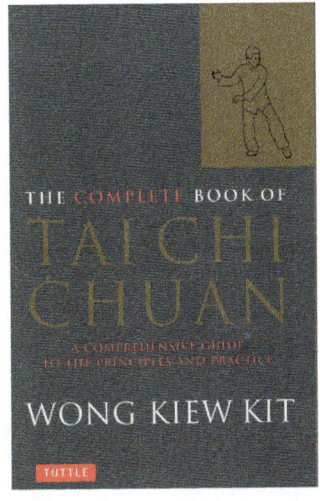

As I've said elsewhere in these reviews, my comments on or criticisms of Taiji literature should not extend to my impression of the author's personal expertise in Taiji. I've seen better books by lesser practitioners and lesser books by acknowledged and high-level experts. According to the blurb on the back cover of Wong Kiew Kit's *The Complete Book of Tai Chi Chuan*, the author has practiced and taught Shaolin arts for more than thirty years and has more than 2,000 students. He has an excellent lineage and has written several other books on the martial arts. His postures in the photos look great, and I have no reason to doubt his abilities or knowledge in the least. In fact, I was looking forward to reading this book, though as soon as I began, I immediately found myself annoyed with the author. The book begins thus:

> Tai Chi Chuan, or Taijiquan in Romanized Chinese, is a wonderful art, but more than 90 per cent of these who practice it gain less than 10 per cent of its potential benefits! This book will not only justify this claim, but will also provide the information you need to gain the remaining 90 per cent of the benefits.

A writer who commits to sweeping claims right at the outset should make every effort to deliver the goods. In the end, Wong does not, though this book does contain a few gems hidden in the tangle. Let's take his opening lines, quoted above. The gem, though not unfamiliar, is the claim that Taiji "is a wonderful art." But all that business about the percentage of people who "don't get it" is unsubstantiated despite the exactness of his figures. And the ideas that this chapter will justify that claim and cure all your Taiji ills are not born out in the least.

At bottom, *The Complete Book of Tai Chi* is a marginally adequate, if sometimes misleading overview of Taiji geared for beginners. Wong opens with a preface in which he makes several statements, such as:

> If a student who has patiently practiced Tai Chi Chuan for many years still remains sickly, weak, emotionally unstable or mentally dull, then he or she has not been judicious or wise. Such a person should either turn to something else, or seek more information from masters or books to improve his or her practice. Generally, people who have correctly practiced an established method for a year should reap the benefits that method is reputed to bring.

This statement plays on the old Taiji saw that says: If you don't practice correctly, then you will miss your mark, and all your practice will have been in vain. In general, I take exception with this idea. Perhaps it is true that if you don't practice correctly or fully—with intent, internal energy, etc.—then you will not become a proficient martial artist or manipulator of chi. I do agree in principle with this idea, but the truth is, most people who practice Taiji don't want to become masters. They just want a healthy exercise that is interesting and has many practical and beneficial results, and Taiji can deliver those even if you don't practice it martially. But according to the old saw, they should abandon even that if they are not dedicated to reaching the top of the Taiji mountain.

Wong, however, takes the idea of deficiency to a new level that borders on the absurd. I've watched a lot of people come to Taiji, and while a few stayed, many of them left. These numbers were mostly made up of relatively healthy and stable people—normal people—with a scattering of "sickly, emotionally unstable, weak or mentally dull" in the mix. The truth is, people with these unfortunate characteristics are, for the most part, constitutionally incapable of going beyond a few lessons.

The notion that such people might actually practice for years—putting out great effort and occupying substantial time yet achieving no results—is absurd. It is true that I've seen people who've practiced for years without martial content whose Taiji is not at all suited for fighting, but even so, it has helped keep them fit, flexible, and focused. It's all in what you want to get out of Taiji and what you're willing to put into it. There is a whole range from absolute beginner to accomplished master, and while one might be able to objectively judge the relative quality of a practitioner's Taiji, one might more profitably consider how nice it is that the amateur practices at all. A Sunday painter's landscape might not be a Gainsborough, but it was a worthy effort for the painter. We all do what we can with what we have to work with.

And the last statement in Wong's paragraph above is equally off the mark. One year of practice will allow you to reap all of Taiji's benefits? What happened to the "kung fu" of Taiji, meaning "excellence gained over time through effort and experience?" I don't know about you, but after only one year, I could perform the form, but I didn't know much of anything about Taiji—how deep it is, how expansive, and how refined it can become.

Chapter one begins:

> Tai Chi Chuan…is one of the most wonderful martial arts in the world. This chapter explains why; so if you are not getting the best from your Tai Chi practice you will at least know what you are lacking.

So he opens the same gem with which he opened his preface, dimming its luster. In fulfilling the part of the statement that reads, "This chapter explains why," the author relies on a general explanation of the differences between hard and soft—or rather, external and internal—martial arts. It's an okay explanation, and to the author's credit, he pens some words of wisdom about the differing psychologies of each approach.

As for the second part, consider that this chapter is only six pages long. That should tell you something about how much Wong can say about "what you are lacking." By the time I reached the chapter's end, the only thing I'd found lacking was a statement on or explanation of what it was that I was lacking.

You know how in a bad movie someone will say something or something will happen that makes you laugh aloud at its unwitting absurdity? Well consider this:

> You can, for example, have a morning walk in the park wearing your business suit, practice your Tai Chi Chuan without attracting the embarrassing attention from uninvited spectators, which is often accorded to other martial arts, and then go straight to your office.

Can you really practice Taiji in a public park while wearing a business suit and not attract attention? When I do Taiji in the park, I attract attention while wearing sweats. And I'd certainly stare with a bemused smile at some guy doing Taiji in a business suit, though I'd probably be more interested in what style he was performing.

Later, Wong writes:

> Just 15 minutes a day in the comfort of your home can provide you with all the exercise you need but can find neither the time nor the energy for.

First of all, fifteen minutes a day is not nearly enough, even for Taiji. It it often said that to become reasonably proficient at Taiji, you have to practice at least an hour a day, and if you want to attain mastery, you have to practice all day, as if it's your job. Plus, if you don't have fifteen minutes or enough energy to practice some other form of exercise, then you don't have fifteen minutes to practice Taiji.

The reader might think I'm nitpicking here, but I see this claim of being able to gain health, well-being, and martial proficiency with minimal time and effort to be the same old misleading claim often used to suck in those who want a quick and easy fix to their problems. They are drawn like moths to the flame of Taiji, only to find that the flame is but the glitter of an imaginary place where one can trade a little for a lot. The truth is, energy cannot be created or destroyed, but it can be transformed. That's what exercise does. It transforms the exerciser from one energy state to another, and to claim that Taiji is some sort of perpetual motion machine that requires no input to reap an output is false advertising. The smoothness and purposefulness of a Taiji player's movements are neither congenital nor magical. Taiji, even at the middling levels, takes work, dedication, and thought, and while teachers and writers should not endeavor to frighten away prospective practitioners by emphasizing those aspects, those aspects need to be faced, not glossed over.

Chapter two continues with these sorts of extravagant and erroneous statements:

> Not one of the more than a dozen English Tai Chi Chuan books I found in a recent survey provides any substantial information on the martial aspects of the system, although most of those written in Chinese describe it as a martial art.

Huh? Well, of course Chinese books on Taiji would acknowledge it as a martial art. But what about those in English? Wong surveyed "more than a dozen" and found no information on Taiji as a martial art? I'm not sure what books he looked at, but as of the writing of his book in 2002, there were hundreds of books in English on Taiji by acknowledged masters who discussed it as a martial art, complete with illustrations of how it can be used in practical situations and some level of detail on push hands. Don't believe me? Check out the other reviews in this series. Yang Jwing-ming, for example, was even then a prolific author on Taiji's use as a martial art, and there were many, many dozens of others—some writing original works and some providing English translations of the Chinese works Wong alludes to.

Not everything in this book is questionable. In relating the history of Taiji, Wong does not resort to the evocative yet simplistic story of Chang Sanfeng. Instead he gives an alternate history of the art's foundation in Taoism and genesis in the Wudang Mountains. Chang comes in later, as do other legendary and almost mythic figures of Taiji, leading up to the art's codification in Chen Village. It's a different history than most, and who knows? Maybe he's right. But it really makes me wish that some trained historian would produce a definitive and detailed history of Taiji, despite the fact that the art seems to have little in the way of evidence from times prior to its nominal inception in Chen Village. The chapter finishes with an adequate history of the development of the major modern Taiji styles.

In chapter four, Wong translates and provides commentary to a few of the more venerable of the Taiji Classics. This material is generally well presented and some of the best in the book, though it is brief at eight pages. Chapter five covers basic Taiji principles and mechanics—including a few self-defense maneuvers—and again, the information is adequate and well-explained and is accompanied by a few well-done drawings. Some of these drawings—the figure drawings, especially—are useful, but the foot-stepping diagrams are less so.

One useful addition is a several-page discussion of knee injuries and how to prevent them, but even here, Wong has to make a statement that is not accurate:

> Throughout the long history of Taijiquan and other forms of martial arts in China, knee injury has never been a problem at all.

Really? I remember watching an interview with a veteran Chinese kung fu actress, then in middle age, who loudly bemoaned the damage that martial arts had done to her knees. Knee injury is always a possibility in the martial arts, sports, gymnastics, or any other motion-based activity, including dance. But it's nice to see the issue addressed here since it usually is ignored in most martial arts books.

Chapter six covers the basic concepts of chi kung, internal force, and abdominal breathing without going into a great deal of detail on any of them. Then the author moves on to form. Although he's often negated the importance of form—namely in the persons of those who only practice form and the impossibility of learning form from any source other than a competent teacher—he now expends chapter seven on the "official" 24-Pattern Simplified Taiji Set and the 40-Pattern Simplified Set. The scanty written instructions are accompanied by adequate if small line drawings.

Push hands and combat techniques occupy chapters eight through eleven, and the text is accompanied by well-done line drawings. The techniques are basic, but they do demonstrate push hands mechanics and show how some Taiji movements can be used. "Enriching Daily

Life with Taiji Chuan" is the title of chapter twelve, and the information here—on the basics of traditional Chinese medicine, internal energy, and relaxation—is all okay but rudimentary.

Then, for several chapters, Wong moves more deeply into form. Having already depicted the 24-Pattern and 48-Pattern Simplified Sets, he now presents drawings of six more Taiji forms: Wudang, Chen, Yang, Wu(/Hao) (Wu Yueh-hsiang), Wu (Wu Quanyu), and Sun Styles. These do not have explanatory texts other than form name lists, and they are done very much in a style pioneered in 1980 by Jou Tsung-hwa in his *The Tao of Tai Chi Chuan* (reviewed earlier in this volume), which depicts two Chen forms, Wu Yueh-hsiang's form, and Yang Style in the same manner. The characteristics of these various forms are recognizable to more experienced practitioners, but they probably would go right over the heads of most beginners if these drawings were all they had to go by. However, when Wong's book came out, these charts were probably more useful than they are now since static depictions of form have been eclipsed by *YouTube* videos of everybody from great masters to average players displaying martial arts forms of nearly every sort and caliber. So I have to give Wong credit here for recording things worth recording at the time.

Chapter nineteen covers weapons, and again, the information is okay but rudimentary. The final two chapters discuss Taiji philosophy and Taoism, often playing off the Taiji Classic and the *Tao Te Ching*. As before, the information is adequate but basic.

I've been hard on this author, but his language—and even ideas—frequently grated on me. All too often, his interpretation of received Taiji wisdom is packaged—embedded—in an absolutist attitude, such as: If you practice Taiji for years and still can't use it, then your time, your practice, has been wasted. Benefits don't always entail use. I personally believe that adding martial intent to the movements adds greater dimension to Taiji, but I've also seen that just doing the form improves muscle tone, encourages joint flexibility, and limbers tendons, even for those who are not martially inclined and never plan to use the movements to fight. After all, the effects of aging are the enemies we all must battle as long as we live. That is the real enemy that Taiji combats.

At the same time, I did read a few nuggets of knowledge and wisdom in these pages, though they could not, in the end, outweigh my annoyance. Ironically, the most pertinent and lasting part of this book is not all the verbiage by Wong, who several times early in the text casts aspersions on the possibility of learning Taiji from a book, but its depiction of the various forms. Even if this sort of material has been superseded by *YouTube*, it wasn't at the time, and it's worthy of being recorded.

In the end, though, I have to say that this book is not the "complete book," it professes to be, and in fact, it is less informative than a great number of other Taiji overviews.

The Big Book of Tai Chi
Build Health Fast in Slow Motion

by Bruce Frantzis
(Blue Snake Books, 1998, 2007, 396 pages)

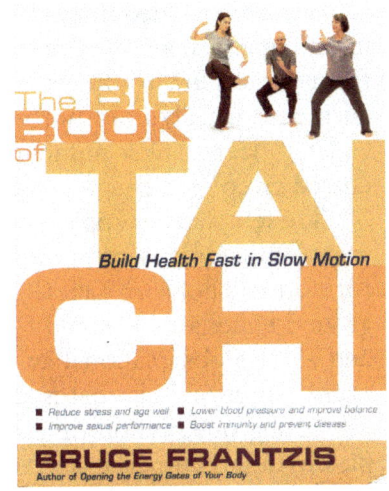

In order to characterize Bruce Frantzis's *The Big Book of Tai Chi*, I have to lead off with two different concepts. The first, which is stated in the book's subtitle, is "slow motion." Taiji is a movement art that is generally practiced at speeds slower than one would usually move. There are a great many reasons to practice Taiji slowly, one of which is that it enables the practitioner to more carefully observe the physicality, balance, flow, and dynamics of the various movements. In other words, practicing at slow speeds allows the practitioner to relax and have greater time for observational awareness.

Tied to slow speed and observational awareness is the idea of mental discipline. As with slowness, there are many aspects to this idea, but pertinent at the moment is that Taiji's slow speed encourages one to slow down and sublimate the overt conscious thinking process. This helps one loosen the inhibitory control over one's movements that is created by the constant stream of conscious thoughts running through our heads. If one thinks ten thoughts while performing a movement at normal speeds, then one will think one hundred thoughts while performing the same movement at one-tenth normal speed. Over time, moving slowly aids one in learning to slow down and ignore the constant chatter in one's head and focus even more deeply on observational awareness.

The second concept is linked to my general definition of beginner's manuals, which usually are manuals for those interested in taking up Taiji or those who have only recently begun practicing. These books are all very similar, generally leading off with some background material which includes history, philosophy, operational precepts, health effects, and other matters, such as how to find a teacher. Then there comes a long section detailing a Taiji form—usually consisting of photos accompanied by instructional text. Next there sometimes are demonstrations of push hands and applications for the moves. And finally, sometimes, a few of the Taiji Classics are included in the body text after the instruction section or in an appendix. In such books, the background material can range from the shallow to the profound, but no matter how well presented it is, it usually does not go into great detail on any one subject and will leave out a number of topics that could be further discussed given greater space.

These concepts apply to *The Big Book of Tai Chi* in a very Taiji way. Although it is, in some ways, a beginner's book, there are no form instructions or Taiji Classics. Instead, Frantzis takes the background material one would find in a beginner's book, slows it down and applies observational awareness to completely parse just about every aspect of Taiji that is not directly related to form. It's sort of like taking one section of a Taiji form, slowing it down, and completely describing each and every aspect and movement, from the macro to the micro. In essence, he's taken material that most Taiji authors present in, say, thirty pages, and slowed it down ten times to fill three hundred pages, revealing details that the others have glossed over or ignored entirely.

The results are curious in a way that has nothing to do with the information itself, the manner of its presentation, or the writing, which is authoritative and more than adequate in terms of style. The oddness comes from trying to figure out just who the audience is. At the beginning of the book, an author's note reads:

> My purpose is to share ideas about how and why tai chi works to stimulate thought and further inquiry. My experience of studying in China for 11 years with masters in tai

chi and chi gung has given me a unique perspective. I hope this book will encourage scientists to make formal studies of tai chi's health benefits, inspire people to try tai chi, and provide tools to enable current tai chi practitioners and instructors to upgrade their skills and gain more benefits and satisfaction from their practice.

I think that Frantzis succeeds in addressing some of these matters—particularly the latter two—but he is less successful with others. On the surface, this book is sort of like a very thick advertising brochure that tries to convince a prospective buyer of a product or service to buy this particular one. It is a raison d'être for taking up Taiji, and the material it presents is as deep as it is voluminous. But I have to wonder just how many people shopping for Taiji are apt to buy and read a three-hundred-page book prior to signing up for a class. In my experience, most people approach Taiji by seeking a local instructor rather than by reading books about it first, though I have to admit that once I decided to take up Taiji, I read a couple of books on it during the interval between signing up and attending the first class. But I'm a voracious reader. *The Big Book of Tai Chi* is a lot of book to read for someone just thinking about taking Taiji.

Worse, while Frantzis touts the great many benefits of Taiji practice—and does so well—he also makes learning Taiji seem like a daunting task. Okay, it is, but at beginner levels, the difficulties are generally physical and rather basic. So when Frantzis starts talking about having to learn material like the 16-Part Nei Gung system and other aspects that are more of a concern to intermediate and advanced students and that obviously take years, if not decades, of practice, I wonder if he makes the Taiji learning curve seem too steep for the average person. This is sort of ironic, considering that the book's subtitle is "Build Health Fast in Slow Motion." You can't build anything if you discourage the builders from participating, and further, you can't really build Taiji fast. Taiji is all about slow, from the speed of the movements to the length of time required to master the basic tenets and onward to progressively greater skill and understanding.

Although the book's obvious target audience seems to be folks shopping for Taiji, at the same time, the pages contain a lot of information that would be more of of interest to intermediate and more advance practitioners, who don't seem to be the overt target audience. Unlike a lot of Western teachers of the internal martial and exercise arts, Frantzis spent some time learning from experts in China, and he possesses a lot of information that is not common knowledge among Western Taiji practitioners. And a lot of that knowledge has found its way into this book, though it is interspersed with a great deal of information that would be well known to the average Taiji journeyman. And as for this book inspiring scientists to study Taiji, well, they'd have to read it first, and it doesn't seem like the sort of book the average researcher might pick up to gain inspiration. But I say this while being a lover of scientific research into Taiji and related internal arts.

Okay, now down to the nuts-and-bolts of the book. We already know that *The Big Book of Tai Chi* is not an instruction manual. Nor is it an intensive look at principles, though many principles and precepts are covered to a greater or lesser extent. Instead, it is a low-altitude and very thorough survey of the Taiji landscape, and you are given a picture of the broader view as well as more sharply focused examinations of specific important features of the terrain.

The book opens with a lengthy introduction by Diane Rappaport, one of Frantzis's more senior students. Then Frantzis takes over, defining Taiji in chapter one. This includes definitions of chi, Taoist energy arts, and other basic information. Chapter two delves into the background of traditional Chinese medicine. It is a detailed overview that includes discussions of the meridian system, the philosophy behind traditional Chinese medicine, and several types of health: physical, emotional, psychological, and spiritual.

Chapter three is on how Taiji improves health, and it includes several specific exercises for strengthening the legs and stances. Twisting, turning, and spiraling are discussed, as are alignments, relaxation, and increasing chi flow. Chapter four discusses how Taiji helps reduce and manage stress. Taiji and longevity is the subject of chapter five, and here Frantzis devotes considerable space to practitioners who are older than fifty. Taiji's benefits for different groups of people occupy chapter six. One focus here is how Taiji can benefit office workers, and another is how it benefits people with disabilities.

Chapter seven discusses Taiji for physical and emotional self-defense, but don't expect attack-and-response photos, though there are a handful. Instead, Frantzis explores the differences between the internal and external martial arts, the stages of learning Taiji as a martial art, practicing with weapons, and push hands. Taiji and spirituality are covered in the next chapter, and the material here frequently becomes more philosophical in content. Some of the topics are meditation, dissolving energy blockages, and connecting one's essence to the Tao.

Choosing a Taiji style is covered in chapter nine, and while this might seem like beginner material, Frantzis uses the space to discuss the major Taiji styles and their differences, large frame versus short frame styles, long forms versus short forms, and the best style for a beginner based on the person's individual needs and desires. It's a very nice summation, and the information is useful for anyone pondering which style to follow or those wanting to know a little bit about styles other than their own.

Frantzis uses these ideas to segue into chapter ten, which discusses what a beginner can expect to learn, Taiji's several levels of complexity, challenges to learning, and learning strategies. He continues in this same vein in chapter eleven, now targeting what intermediate and advanced students can expect to learn. This is all useful information for teachers as well as students. One facet of learning is integrating the Three Treasures: body, energy, and spirit. He also talks about how to transition from external to internal movements, coordinating movement with breath, circularity, five progressive stages of twisting and spiraling, chi development, fa jin, and how to practice for high-level performance. A subsection describing the Taiji Classics is included, but Frantzis does not replicate any of the Classics themselves.

Choosing a teacher is the subject of the final chapter. After this are three appendices: on the differences between Taiji and chi kung, on the Five Elements, and on the differences between Taiji and yoga.

I do have to mention one production flaw in this book. The type font used for the body text is a sanserif. For those who don't know, a serif font has little ticks, called serifs, at the end of each line, like the typeface used in this book. Sanserif fonts don't—"san" means "without." This is an F in a serif font, and this is an F in a sanserif font. In printed pieces, serif fonts help the eye distinguish the various characters more readily than do fonts without serifs. Typographers generally agree that sanserif fonts do not work well for large amounts of body text in printed works. Serf fonts are much better for that, while sanserif fonts are generally relegated to miscellaneous copy: headlines, subheads, sidebars, and captions for photos and illustrations. Oddly, just the opposite is true of web pages, where, for some reason, sanserif fonts tend to work better than serif fonts for body text. Maybe that's because serifs in large amounts of body copy on a screen make text look "heavy." Unfortunately, the body copy in *The Big Book of Tai Chi* is set in a sanserf font that also is fairly light in weight. Maybe the book designer thought that the light sanserif font was an elegant touch, but reading this lengthy book was a chore for my eyesight. Typography should aid in reading, not inhibit the process.

I've glossed over a great deal of what this book has to offer since Frantzis goes into depth as well as breadth that is not easily or succinctly summarized. You'll have to read the book to get all the details. But I will say that *The Big Book of Tai Chi*, though unusual in some respects, is basically a nuts-'n-bolts book that eschews form instruction and tries to get at the base ground of what Taiji is and how it works. It's well written, informative, and covers some material not easily found elsewhere. It's not a must, perhaps, but it would be a valuable addition to any Taiji library.

Genuine Explanations for Authentic Tai Chi

By Wu Zhiqing
(Originally published by Great East Bookstore, 1936. B*rennan Translations*, 2016, 264 pages.)

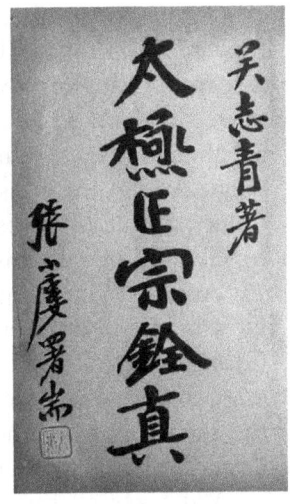

Wu Zhiqing, the author of *Genuine Explanations for Authentic Tai Chi*, is a mystery to me. I was unable to find anything on him aside from this book and the few brief autobiographical statements it contains. Wu was from Guxi, in Anhui, and he met Yang Chengfu in 1918 and began studying with him. "I practiced day and night, making a thorough study of it." This lasted "for several years," and the author also talks about reading and learning from Sun Lutang's *A Study of Taiji Boxing*, Chu Minyi's *Taiji Boxing Photographed*, and Chen Weiming's *The Art of Taiji Boxing*. "I pondered their contents until I deeply understood." Certainly these were learned Taiji practitioners who produced excellent and informative books that any Taiji student should one day read and think about.

The structure of most Taiji manuals—and martial arts manuals in general—goes like this:

1) Prefaces and/or Introductions
2) Introductory material, such as history, philosophy, and methodology
3) Form instruction—photographs with text, and occasionally, foot-stepping charts

4) Push hands, sparring, and application instruction
5) A sampling—sometimes extensive—of quotes from the Taiji Classics
6) Ancillary material, such as appendices, index, bibliography, and even self-promotional material

Sometimes elements are missing or the order is mixed up, but this is the basic structure. Wu mixes it up in a couple of unexpected ways. First, his sketchy introductory sections on history, philosophy, and methodology are dispensed with in a total of only four pages. About half a page of this is repetition, and a full page is a discussion of the numbering and naming conventions of Taiji movements.

As far as numbering goes, Wu points out that the number of movements any give Taiji form contains is a deceptive way to define a form. A single movement in one form might be enumerated as more than one in another, even while the dynamics and purpose(s) are the same. For example, in some styles, Grasping Bird's Tail and Single Whip are considered to be one entire movement, while in others, Single Whip is a movement distinct from, though attached to, Grasping Bird's Tail.

And as any Taiji practitioner knows, the names of similar movements in different forms sometimes vary: Grasping Bird's Tail, Grasping Sparrow's Tail, Catch the Sparrow by the Tail, etc., for example. And there are names that are completely different though the movement are the same. Sun Lutang calls the first movement Grand Polarity rather than the more common Preparation.

Wu takes all this a valuable step farther by providing a seven-page comparative list of four Yang Taiji forms—those practiced by Chen Weiming, Sun Lutang, Chu Minyi, and the author. Chen is widely considered one of Yang Chengfu's premier students and was the founder of a number of important Taiji schools and academies. Sun Lutang is most famous for being an internal style syncretist. And Chu Minyi, a Wu stylist, also was a leading figure in the Chinese Republican movement and early Nationalist government as well as an important martial arts author.

While Wu is light on discussions of precepts and methodology, what advice he does give tends to be good and adequately stated—even containing occasional kernels of wisdom:

> For any who practice boxing arts, an understanding of how to use hand, eye, body, technique, and stepping is the the basic course of training.... For your hands to attack, your body to evade, or your steps to suit your advancing, always use stepping as the standard. That is why every boxing set pays attention to how the feet are positioned and how directions are faced.

In other words, heavy on bottom, light on top, yet agile throughout, or, if there is error, seek first to correct the feet and legs.

I also like it that the author frequently distinguishes Taiji not by its practice speed, but by its characteristic of smooth continuity. But consider, now, his oddly reasoned argument concerning the then-prevailing question of which style is "authentic": Chen or Yang. This might seem to be a somewhat ridiculous disagreement to those of us today who have clear historical references to resolve the matter, but Wu enters into it anyway. Perhaps being that close to Taiji's early days rendered its origins somewhat more opaque—a problem that has since been resolved by documentation. (Though fanatics continue to introduce alternative histories. Do disinformation, misinformation, and malinformation comprise the real plague of our time?)

In any event, Wu comes down on the side of the Chens, but not for the historical reason you might assume. Being a direct student of Yang Chengfu and thus relatively close to the origins of Yang Style Taiji, surely he'd heard Yang family lore, which would have included the fact that Yang Luchan—only two generations removed—learned Taiji from the Chen family.

Yet instead of resorting to that simple historical fact, Wu utilizes an elaborate argument based on the evolution over time of Taiji's naming conventions. When I first read this argument, I was puzzled at why Wu bothered. But as I better understood his book, I realized that what I had seen as pointless argument had really been part of the fabric of Wu's efforts to fashion a new sort of Taiji book. That will become more clear as we go on to look at Wu's form instruction section, which follows the brief introductory material.

He titles this section, Part One, and quite a section it is, occupying two hundred pages. It depicts, the author says, a Yang Style that he learned to from Yang Chengfu, seasoned with material from Chen Weiming and Sun Lutang. The form consists of eighty-one named movements, which, thanks to the form comparison chart, can be compared to the forms of Chen Weiming, Sun Lutang, and Chu Minyi. All-in-all, the form instruction section is adequate, with decent descriptions and photos that, while a little dull to the eye, have enough contrast to recognize what Wu is doing and to see the directional arrows embedded in the photos. A scattering of helpful footwork charts completes the form instruction section.

The next major section of the book, Part Two, contains several essays that discuss various aspects of Taiji. They are not authored by Wu, however, but by various Taiji experts, most notably the aforementioned Chen Weiming. Some of these essays tackle practical aspects, such as precepts and principles, others are more politically oriented—for example, the first chapter is Hu Pu'an's, "The Value of Taiji Boxing in Physical Education" (from *Eastern Variety Magazine*, Vol. 30, #20, October 1933). Hu begins with an explanation—one among many out there in the world—of how Taiji acquired its name. His discussion takes into account Taiji's energy dynamics, which are centered in the tantien.

> The universe is a grand polarity, and the human body is also a grand polarity. The belly represents the grand polarity, the two sides of the waist represent the dual aspects, the two arms and two legs represent the four manifestations, and the upper and lower sections of each limb represent the eight trigrams. The motive power of the universe lies in the Grand Polarity, and the motive power of the human body also lies in a grand polarity. Therefore the movements in Taiji Boxing are not the movements of the hands and feet, but the movement of the waist, and not really even the waist, but the abdomen.

Next, under the heading, "Taiji Boxing's Movements," Hu goes into several foundational Taiji precepts: "Your body should be loose," "Your energy should be firm," and "Your spirit should be concentrated." Each aspect is treated to an explanation. Then comes a slightly longer subsection on the subject of the title of this chapter.

The next chapter encompasses material from Jiang Rongqiao's "Annotations to Wang Zongyue's [Wang Tseung-yueh] Taiji Boxing Treatise," which was originally included in *Taiji Boxing Explained* (1930), by Jiang Rongqiao and Yao Fuchun. At twenty-three pages, this is easily the longest chapter in Part Two, but I'm not going to discuss the content here except to say that it is all worthwhile material from two excellent writers. The reason I'm not going into this section is that I reviewed that book elsewhere in this volume. If you have not read the original—or even if you have—this material is excellent and wide-ranging.

Next is "Yang Chengfu's Ten Essentials of Taiji Boxing," from Chen Weiming's *Art of Taiji Boxing* (1925). (Reviewed in Volume VI of this series.) If there are ten essentials to Taiji, these are them, handed down by one of the premier names of the art. Each is accompanied by explanatory text.

A couple of essays by Sun Lutang follow, from his *A Study of Taiji Boxing* (1921). (Sun's book is discussed in Volume IV of this series.)

This segues into Chen Zhijin's essay, "Taiji Boxing's Moral Qualities and Functions," the original of which appeared in Chen Weiming's *Taiji Sword* (1928). (Reviewed in Volume IV of this series.) This essay begins with a somewhat lengthy and apocryphal telling of the Zhang (Chang) Sanfeng legend, then states that there are three strict moral rules to practicing the martial arts:

1) I cannot become a bodyguard, protecting caravans and courtyards.
2) I cannot become a street performer, making money off its exhibition.
3) I cannot become an outlaw hiding in the forest.

Translator Paul Brennan humorously clarifies these in this way:

> In other words, the purpose of this stuff is not to enable you to become a cop, a movie star, or a criminal.

The first, at least, however, is curious since it's no secret that some of the patriarchs of both the Yang and Wu families (Yang Banhao, Wu Quanyu, and Wu Chienchuan, for example) were high-ranking bodyguards for Manchurian royalty. And certainly, the third prohibition would be moot to anyone engaged in criminal activity, entailing the necessary violation of the first by those seeking to stop the criminals—and the subsequent idolizing of the first by the second. Martial arts performance, whether in the street, in the theater, in film, or on TV, has been a staple of the martial arts from time immemorial. We're still little more than cavemen reenacting visions of victories before the flickering and unsure light of the campfire. For people to stop telling martial arts tales is about as likely as it is for criminals to stop criming and for cops to stop pursuing them.

Another set of prohibitions in Chen's essay also are amusing. Do not gnash your teeth or stare hard with your eyes. (Okay, but it's kind of hard to do either if you're relaxed enough to be doing Taiji, though I once witnessed a man doing Taiji whose eyes literally blazed with madness.) Do not shout aggressively or make strange cries. (Hear that, Bruce Lee?) And most amusingly, "when practicing the solo set, you cannot be naked." (I guess nobody told that to Martin Sheen in *Apocalypse Now*, William Sadler in *Die Hard 2*, or Patrick Swayze in *Road House*. But then, the first two were basically bad guys, and Patrick was the good guy, so he was wearing pants.) (I also have to wonder at the true function of this since all of us are, at all times, naked beneath our clothing.) (And finally, I would be remiss if I didn't note the book, *Tai Chi Nude* by F. L. Yu, reviewed in Volume VI of this series.)

The final essay is "Chen Weiming's Experience of Teaching Taiji Boxing." There is no citation for this essay, so I assume it was original to this book. It is only a single page and does not really address the subject of its title in any significant way. Chen mostly lays out several Taiji principles, some with thumbnail descriptions, some not. He finishes the essay with a couple of two-line, un-resourced anecdotes about miraculous cures of temperament and irritability effected by Taiji. Okay, but that's it.

This book is worthwhile in a couple of aspects, and less so in others. Let's take a look at the deficits first, because the assets are so much more valuable and significant. The dearth of text by the author is both a deficit and a benefit. On the deficit side, one could argue that this book isn't really by Wu, which is true since he wrote only the form instruction section and almost nothing on all those important aspects of Taiji besides form instruction that are normally covered. While it's not unusual for a Taiji book to contain chapters by other authors—or from the Taiji Classics—usually those are added to embellish the author's own text, not to entirely substitute for it.

But maybe it's a good thing that Wu let others speak for him. His Taiji skills might be significant, but his writing skills are, shall we say, not up to the task of authoring an entire, in-depth book about Taiji. "I am not very bright," he admits. "but I did learn Taiji Boxing from Yang Chengfu for several years."

Well, he's bright enough to have taken the expert instruction in Taiji that he received and become relatively expert. So the one place his writing does excel is in the lengthy form instruction section, where the descriptions are generally neat and clear. But the mercifully short opening sections where he introduces and discusses Taiji are pedantic and crudely and repetitively written and reveal a generally weak writing skill. So it is well that he let those others say what he could not, especially since they were experts influential to his own development as well as better writers.

Another good thing about the inclusion of these other authors is that the reader gets a wider variety of perspectives on the art than usually exists in books by single authors. However, except for a couple of the chapters of Part Two, most of the material is available in its original and more thorough publications. You can find several of them at *Brennan Translations* (https://brennantranslation.wordpress.com), so if you discovered this book there, you can find them, as well, at this valuable resource.

One reason I like writing these reviews is that doing so forces me to take a closer look at texts than I otherwise might. Often that produces no greater insight than what is apparent at first glance because nothing else is to be had. But sometimes, broader or deeper aspects that require some thought to discern are revealed by closer examination. Such was the case with this book.

With that in mind, anyone who has read many of my reviews knows that I'm generally not a fan of form instruction material. Really, how many people ever learned Taiji from a book? Heck, most people can't seem to learn it from a live teacher. But there is something to be said for depictions of the forms of historical practitioners. They can help give a sense of both the development of the art and its inevitable "drift" as it transmutes over time. In other words, in addition to being valuable historical artifacts in their own right, they can help anchor the art's roots in its historical precepts—in this case, a Yang Style learned from Yang Chengfu and closely resembling the one practiced by Chen Weiming, another historically significant figure in the development and dissemination of Taiji.

And this brings us back to the lengthy lists of form movements in the introductory material, as well to Wu's writing on the numbering and naming conventions for the movements—and his seemingly unnecessary argument using those conventions to validate a blatantly obvious historical fact. Perhaps, in true yin/yang sense, his real purpose was actually to validate the usefulness of naming conventions in solving historical and relational issues among the various Taiji styles. In addition, the comparative form list is interesting in its own right, especially to those interested in the development of Yang Style.

So, along with the range of content in Part Two, the gestalt of the book becomes more apparent. This is not an average Taiji manual, though it resembles one and can be seen as and used in that way. Instead, this is one of the earliest examples I know of comparative martial arts scholarship.

Comparative scholarship of this sort was not prevalent in martial arts literature at the time Wu compiled this book. Only in the last half-century has this sort of research into various aspects of the martial arts begun to be explored in significant depth—thanks, in part, to the expansion of the martial arts into the West, where culture exhibits a more analytical mindset. So we have to consider Wu a forerunner of the trend toward research into and analysis of the martial arts—above and beyond form work, sparring, fighting, and so forth. This is especially true given the contents of Part Two, which displays a range of topics, some not usually discussed in martial arts literature.

For the average reader, this book would be of most value to those who have not read the chapters by the other authors in their original publications. The more discursive will find interest in the clues this book contains regarding the development of Yang Style, particularly, as well as of Wu Family Style, considering the Chu Minyi connection. Scholars of martial arts literature should take note of this volume's place on the shelf labeled, "Research."

The YMCA Taiji Boxing Club's Anniversary Book

By the Shanghai YMCA Taiji Boxing Club
(Originally published 1929. *Brennan Translations*, 2017, 50 pages)

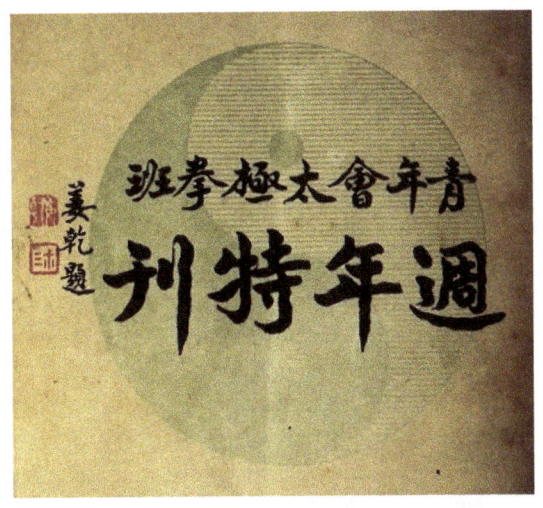

You know you're not in Kansas when the local YMCA has a Taiji boxing club.

The book opens with a group photo of the staff of the YMCA Taiji Boxing Club, though none of the fourteen men are named. Next comes photos of several of them demonstrating twelve isolated Taiji form postures, four push hands postures, and two sword postures. Some of the postures illustrate elements of the Eight Gates, but some are just postures from a Taiji form.

The various chapters of this book were written by different individuals. The text begins with a preface by Peng Yuyi in which he gives a sketchy but adequate history of the club. The next text, by Xie Dexuan, discusses the origins of Taiji. This is the extended version that traces five major origin stories, only one of which involves Chang Sanfeng. I've seen this sort of inclusive rendition of Taiji's origins in half a dozen Chinese martial arts manuals and books, and it warrants further examination since we all know that Chang Sanfeng, even if he existed, could not have been the sole developer of flexible, internal martial arts. The only problem with this section is that Xie gives no dates, though occasionally he mentions the dynasty in which the developments were taking place.

Xie continues with another chapter on how Taiji benefits health, and another on his experience of learning Taiji. Then comes a list of the names of a forty-nine-posture Yang Style form, but just the names—no textual instructions, photos, or illustrations.

Bi Zibi writes the next two short chapters on how he treated his illness by practicing Taiji and his take on perseverance in training. Sheng Xiaoxian comes up next, with a chapter on how practicing Taiji can alter one's state of mind—essential that it can help improve memory and strengthen the will.

Shen Junwen then writes on key to practicing Taiji. This chapter contains ideas about Taiji's learning curve, the mental aspect of the art, using energy appropriately, distinguishing between empty and full, relaxation, and several other important Taiji precepts, all of which he states succinctly but with some thoroughness.

Qiu Zuwang chimes in with his own take on learning Taiji and the benefits that have accrued from his practice, and ditto on the following chapters by Xu Shiyuan, Wang Weichang, Huang Dingliang, and Peng Zunlu. Peng then digresses on his strongly positive feelings regarding the club on its first anniversary.

Next comes a chapter by the notable Chu Minyi in which he discusses Taiji's characteristics. This chapter was mostly excerpted from Chu's own Taiji manual from 1929. (See review in Volume VI of this series.) This is probably one of the strongest chapters in the book, discussing posture, movement, using intention, issuing power, and becoming skillful. Each point is well-dissected by explanatory text.

Provisional rules for the Taiji club end the book. These mostly regard organizational matters.

While this isn't a must-read Taiji book, some of the material—particularly that by Chu Minyi—is worth the effort, though you can find it at greater depth in Chu's own book.

Simple Introduction to Taiji Boxing

By Xu Zhiyi
(Originally published 1927. *Brennan Translations*, 2014, 72 pages)

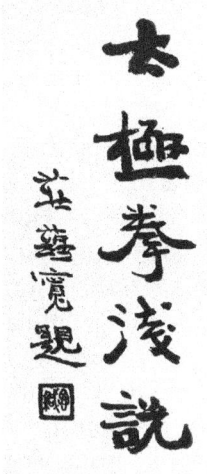

This book on Taiji, by Xu Zhiyi, discusses the art from a Wu Family Style perspective. It isn't a form instruction manual, but rather an overview of the art. A foreword by Gu Xienguang poetically extolls the virtues of the author and the book. This is followed by portraits of Wu Chienchuan and the author, eight Taiji form postures, and the postures of the Eight Gates. The portraits are of decent quality, but not the posture shots.

The author's preface comes next, but it's only about 150 words long and doesn't say much. Nor do the brief general comments that follow or the four prefaces by others that lead into the main text. The first real chapter looks at the origin and development of Taiji. This account begins with the standard Chang Sanfeng story, but it goes into more detail on the post-Chang transmission of the art. Xu names several individuals in the lineage, and even points to a divergence of the art into southern and northern versions—transmitted by Zhang Songzi and Jiang Fa, respectively.

The merits of Taiji boxing are dealt with next. After a brief intro, this section discusses the various aspects of the art:

Health Aspects
 1) It cultivates the mind
 2) The movements are mild.
 3) The postures are smooth and harmonious.

4) Development is natural.
5) It is particularly effective at treating illness.
6) It sculpts your temperament.

Martial Aspects
1) It uses stillness to overcome movement.
2) It uses softness to overcome hardness.
3) It uses the smaller to defeat the larger.
4) It uses smoothness to avoid harm.

Other Aspects
1) Everyone can practice it.
2) It is easy to practice.
3) It is highly enjoyable.

Each of these points is treated to an explanation.

The next chapter is, "Taiji Boxing in Relation to the Study of Psychology." Here, the author discusses Taiji practice as cultivation of both body and mind, thus harmonizing the two and creating a more resilient individual. Sensations and perception are heightened, as is self-examination. He also discusses the right way to study the art—namely by using intention.

Taiji in relation to physiology is the subject of the following chapter, and the several topics discussed in it amount to a number of Taiji principles:

1) Forcelessly press up your head top.
2) Contain your chest, and pluck up your back.
3) Sink your shoulders, and drop your elbows.
4) The Three-Line stance.

Again, each of these elements is explained, and the chapter segues into the next, which deals with Taiji in relation to the study of mechanics. First, Xu discusses how Taiji conforms to Newton's Three Laws of Motion.

> First Law—In the absence of gravity or other external forces, an object in motion tends to remain in motion.

> Second Law—The change of motion of an object is proportional to the force impressed, and is made in the direction of the straight line in which the force is impressed.
>
> Third Law—Every action has an equal and opposite reaction.

He goes over each law, relating it to Taiji, then he examines how Taiji conforms to the principle of net force.

> The original form of Newton's second law states that the net force acting upon an object is equal to the rate at which its momentum changes with time. If the mass of the object is constant, this law implies that the acceleration of an object is directly proportional to the net force acting on the object, is in the direction of the net force, and is inversely proportional to the mass of the object.[1]

Xu writes:

> When using Taiji Boxing to deal with an opponent, it is crucial to avoid going against the direction of his issued energy and resisting it. You should instead yield to the direction of his energy, drawing in his force to land on nothing and thereby causing him to fall into a dangerous position.

More explanations of net force lead into the next chapter, which is on the principle of opposite force. This is a rather complex idea related to Newton's Third Law, entailing the defender to sense the strength and direction of the opponent's force in order to neutralize it or deflect it to the side.

Xu then discusses conforming to the principle of equal force, which he says, causes objects to rotate. The principle of center of gravity comes next, and this concerns finding the greatest stability within one's body.

A discussion of Taiji's practice methods follows, taking into account:

Solo Practice Methods
    1) Awareness and alertness
    2) Connection
        i. Upper body and lower body coordinate

  ii. Inside and out join with each other
  iii. Emptiness and stillness

Partner Practice Methods
 1) Do not crash in.
 2) Do not come away.
 3) Strive at first to open up.
 4) Do not be the first to express power.
 5) Know how to adapt.
 6) Power finishes, but the intent of it continues.

As the author does elsewhere, these point are all explicated.

Chapter eight contains a several-page Q&A that covers a number of interesting and important topics, such as muscle memory, the use of consciousness and intent, being natural, neutralizing energy, and many other valuable points to think about.

That's the end of the main text, which is followed by several appendices. The first consists of several of the Taiji Classics—those supposedly by Chang Sanfeng and Wang Tsungyue. A list of the postures of the Wu Style form that Xu does comes next, but there isn't any instructional text or photos. The penultimate appendix is an essay on the methods of the internal school, written by Huang Baijia, and the final one is a biography of Zhang Songxi, who, the author states, is the progenitor of the southern school of Taiji.

I have to give a thumbs up to this book. Taiji precepts, principles, and methodology are clearly stated, and the book covers a lot of ground, some of which is ignored by other Taiji books. Of special interest is its alternate history of Taiji's development, which warrants further study.

Notes
1 "Force." *Wikipedia*, https://en.wikipedia.org/wiki/Force

Embrace Tiger, Return to Mountain
The Essence of T'ai Chi

By Al Chung-liang Huang
(Real People Press, 1973, 190 pages)

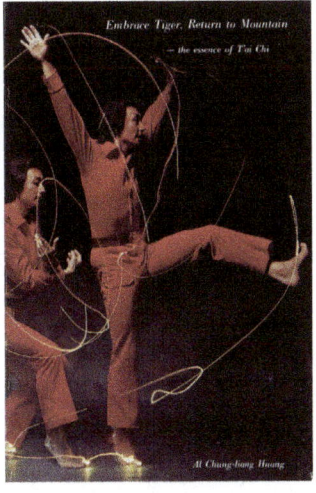

Al Chung-liang Huang, the author of *Embrace Tiger, Return to Mountain: The Essence of T'ai Chi*, enjoys a stellar reputation in many circles, not just Taiji. This from the *Wikipedia* entry on him:

> Chungliang "Al" Huang is a notable philosopher, dancer, performing artist, and internationally acclaimed taijiquan master and educator, having received the Republic of China's most prestigious award in the field of education, the Gold Medal Award, from its Ministry of Education. As the keynote speaker at the Major World Gatherings in India, Switzerland, Germany, and Bali, Chungliang "Al" Huang appeared with many notable world leaders of religion and spiritual philosophy including the Dalai Lama. Huang is the founder-president of the Living Tao Foundation based on the Oregon coast of the United States, and the International Lan Ting Institute, located in the sacred mountains of China. Huang was featured in the inaugural segment of Bill Boyer's renowned PBS series *A World of Ideas*.
>
> Throughout his career, Huang established many close alliances with highly regarded philosophers and scholars of

our time, notably, his colleague and collaborator, the late philosopher scholar Alan Watts, mythologist Jospeh Campbell, and his mentor John Blofeld. He has taught at the Esalen Institute in Big Sur, CA, since the late 1960s.

In addition to associating closely with the above mentioned people, Huang also has been a colleague and collaborator with Laura Huxley, Gregory Batson, Huston Smith, and a host of well-known philosophers, artists, entertainers, and other notables.

This is a pretty heady crowd, and one would expect a great deal from one so highly placed and regarded. Here's a quote from Alan Watts' foreword to the book:

> With his skill in t'ai chi, as well as dancing and flute playing, Huang Chung-liang woos and beguiles his students instead of forcing them. This is the mark of a truly superior and gifted teacher who works upon others as the sun and rain upon plants.

Indeed, Huang seems like a knowledgable, generous, and pleasant man with a large spirit, and I wanted to like his book. Yes, I wanted to like this book, but I utterly hated it.

Born in Shanghai in the 1930s, Huang moved with his family to Taiwan after the end of China's civil war. Throughout his childhood, he studied Taiji with various people, some masters, some just the farmer down the road. In addition to studying the martial arts, he also studied the Classics, fine arts, and Beijing Opera techniques. He moved to the United States in the 1960s to study architecture, cultural anthropology, and choreography. Since then, he has made his living as a Taiji master, a teacher of dance, and a lecturer and teacher of philosophy.

This is not a usual sort of Taiji book, even for one that does not discuss form but focuses instead on principles, philosophy, history, and so forth. This book is basically a faux week-long Taiji workshop cobbled together from several such actual events—primarily from one Huang led at the Esalen Institute in July 1971 that was later edited and embellished with material from other workshops. The book very much reflects its genesis as a workshop rather than as a created text. In other words, the entire book consists of Huang talking to you as if you were participating in the workshop. In principle, this might sound interesting and useful, but in practice is is not.

The problem is two-fold. First, Huang obviously demonstrates much of what he talks about while he's talking, and the reader gets none of that. All we get are words without accompanying photos to visually demonstrate the movements and exercises he's showing the students at the workshop. While it might be possible to follow along with some of his instructions to, in an ersatz way, "participate" in the workshop, most are not that well described or seem kind of pointless—or even impossible—to do on one's own.

Second—and far more egregious from my perspective—is that the Taiji Huang offers is very much a New Age version, with all the namby-pamby baggage involved in that mindset. For Huang, everyone desires to open to experiences and to each other, but that is patently not the case with humankind. The world is filled with unrepentantly evil and egregiously cruel and willfully ignorant people, and to expect them to yearn for goodness and truth is foolishness of the worst sort.

Worse, this mindset leads Huang to make statements about Taiji that either stretch credulity or are factually and dynamically incorrect. For Huang, Taiji is complete freedom. His objective is to let go of all tension and to relax into a oneness with the reality all around. Okay, I can get behind that. He starts by giving a version of that old transcendental tale of the man of knowledge who approaches the spiritually wise master, who then complains that the knowledgable man's cup is already full, so how can he give him anything? It's a wise story, but not when it leads to such open-endedness that it becomes pointless. Will the knowledgeable man, once his cup has been emptied and refilled by the master, have to once again empty his cup? Why, sure.

Huang believes—or seems to—that everything is Taiji and Taiji is everything. Perhaps everything is a mixture of yin and yang and therefore partakes of tai chi (the supreme ultimate), but not everything is the art of Taiji. He even makes a point of saying that he's teaching Taiji, not Taijiquan, because adding the "chuan" part automatically limits the "Taiji" part to its fighting aspect. That is simply not true, and if it were, would the reverse be true, as well? The problem is that he constantly conflates the art of Taiji with the reality behind the philosophy represented by the taijitu, and thus he's not really talking about the art but about the philosophy. Except when he insists that he's talking about the art, anyway.

Huang is so into the so-called freedom he espouses that he fails to realize that when everything is everything, there are no definers. The Tao might be like that, but this reality certainly isn't. That doesn't stop him, though, from saying that doing the Taiji form is to lock oneself up in a constricting and stultifying pattern of movement that will strip your being of initiative and flexibility.

> There is no use to follow the whole sequence of t'ai chi ch'uan and imitate all the motions. If I saw everybody go out on the deck and do it in unison, I wouldn't say "Bravo!" I would say "How sad." So many people just go through the motions mechanically and thats the end of true creativity. I would be unhappy to see that happening to t'ai chi movement. T'ai chi may look from the outside like a pattern or structure, but what is happening inside the body must be very different. T'ai chi is neither a set structure nor chaos. Not this. Not that. It is a different kind of organization which cannot be known by learning a set of patterned movement.... This kind of teaching seems to me like putting on another straight-jacket. Always you are worrying about what to do next, always thinking.

I have to call bullshit on this. Sure, you have to be open inside when you're doing Taiji, but can a beginner be open to anything about Taiji without practicing it for a while—without doing the patterned movements mechanically until the movements become ingrained, natural, and flowing? Or has Huang forgotten that he wasn't always a Taiji master and that he started out by learning forms? Plus, doing Taiji in a group can bring a whole new energy to each of the participants as they meld into a gestalt of energy. And isn't Huang teaching his workshop to a group, and aren't they doing movements together?

Besides, who is Huang to say that everybody doing Taiji in a group is just mechanically going through the motions? Does he personally have access to the internal states of all Taiji players in the world who sometimes practice in groups? He might be correct in saying that Taiji is not a specific set structure—after all, there are many styles of Taiji, which couldn't be the case if it was a set structure instead of a set of principles and rules. However, no matter which style you practice—or even sometimes embellish or deviate from—Taiji is patterned movement based on those principles and rules, all of which must be adhered to for the movement to fit the definition of Taiji and, eventually, to teach you. Principles and rules may not be not hallmarks of total freedom, but they can be launching pads. In other words, freedom does not come without prior restrictions.

In this vein, let me quote Tem Horwitz and Susan Kimmelman from their book, *Tai Chi Ch'uan: The Technique of Power* (reviewed next):

> Although there are people who teach week-end workshops in Tai Chi, claiming to communicate the quality of the movement without the burden of the form, this is in contradiction of the best of the Tai Chi experience. The discipline is indispensable. Tai Chi's unique strength lies in this integration of form and freedom. (P. 22)

Plus, does Huang not practice the form? Early on, he makes a big deal about learning Taiji from many different people. Did none of them practice and teach him a form? The truth is that practicing the form is what teaches you about Taiji and keeps you strong and supple. You can't just wave your arms around and take random steps and call it Taiji unless you're a master already versed in the art, and in that case, there wouldn't be any randomness involved. Taiji movements have meanings, purposes, and results on many levels: physical, mental, emotional, and spiritual, but none of that happens without practicing a legitimate form.

You might, for a time, be mechanical in your practice and worry about what to do next, but isn't that the case with every new endeavor? Learn a new card game, and you're going to have to constantly think about how the game functions and how to best take advantage of the situation, but with experience over time (kung fu), the plays become automatic. Learning to ride a bike is fraught with incompetence and failure until the rider learns about dynamic balance. Taiji is no different. I think I can safely say that no tyro ever approached any endeavor any time or anywhere, much less Taiji, and instantly was perfect at it. Even Albert Einstein had to learn math, with all of its constraints, to open humanity to the momentous conditions of the seemingly infinite reality surrounding us.

Other of his facts are equally suspect. For example, he says in referring to karate, Aikido, Judo, etc.: "All those Japanese forms of movement and centering are very highly developed forms of t'ai chi." This statement makes me think that he needs a refresher course on martial arts history. Certainly Taiji has been an influence on some of the Japanese martial arts, but most of them did not develop directly from Taiji but rather from Shaolin Kung Fu and indigenous Japanese fighting styles already present on the islands.

Or take Huang's take on music:

> [You] may think that if you just keep working and working to fit into that form that someday you will find the freedom—like practicing piano scales. But think how many people practice scales, and how many Horowitzes or Rubinsteins do we have? Do you really believe that you can become a great artist simply by practice, practice, practice?

Maybe not, but I certainly won't become one if I don't practice, practice, practice. It is impossible for a musician to play set pieces or to improvise until he or she knows and understands the scales to be played, and scales are nothing but form practice, plain and simple. There's a famous quote from concert violinist Jascha Heifetz:

> If I don't practice one day, I know it; two days, the critics know it; three days, the public knows it.

"And how many Horowitzes or Rebinsteins do we have?" Huang asks, as if the answer to Taiji mastery consists of inborn talent and nothing else but "flow." Well, there are a huge number of master pianists. That Huang can only name two is more telling about Huang than it is about master pianists or masters of Taiji. Besides, who says I am interested in becoming the Horowitz of Taiji? Apparently, Huang, himself, occupies that position. I have other aspirations. For me, Taiji is a tool for self development, not an end-all and be-all. I don't expect—or even want—to become a great Taiji master. I don't even want more enlightenment than I now have, which is enough for the time being. I just want a reasonably fulfilling life. But Huang seems to think that I should be as invested in freeform Taiji as he is. This attitude, unfortunately, is too often expressed by masters writing on the martial arts who don't recognize that not all of us are driven toward martial mastery. For us, reasonable expertise is the goal.

Huang has a great reputation for the quality of his Taiji, so let's look at that for a moment. Of course, I haven't seen him perform in person, but this is his book, so I feel safe in relying on his statements and photos in it. For example, Huang says this:

> There are a few movements in t'ai chi that require you to stand on one leg, but basically your weight stays centered between your legs, ready to move in any direction.

Really? The Taiji Classics, the expert authors of thousands of Taiji books, and every single Taiji expert and master I've ever personally met say that one of the major principles of Taiji is not to have your weight centered but have it anywhere from 70%/30% to100%/0%. Having the weight evenly distributed is the fault of double-weighting and is a Taiji no-no because it not only inhibits rapid stepping, but also will not allow for the direct transference of energy up the active leg, through the hips and waist, and up the torso into the arms, giving Taiji its whipping quality.

Huang exacerbates the error a couple of pages later, saying:

> When you have your base a little wider, you can shift your weight more easily.

This is simply not true. A wide base require more movement to shift the weight or step out of than a narrow base. Don't believe me? Get in a deep horse stance and move out of it, then try a narrower base. One indisputable fact of the physical world is that small things move more rapidly than large things. A spider can almost instantly leap tens of times farther than the width of its stance, while an elephant can't leap at all. A tiger can move extremely rapidly, but it can't catch the flea hopping and crawling around in its fur.

Some times, Huang just seems pedantic.

> If you understand the principles of the movement, you will not get stuck in worrying about the irrelevant details—how large it should be, or exactly when to begin turning, etc. If you only pay attention to details, you will feel awkward and confined. The minute you feel confined and you stop to think, then the flow get stagnant and polluted. Pretty soon your movement becomes dead and looks as if you are only trying to copy the master' instructions.

Again, this is a pretty irrelevant statement that banks on New Age nonsense. Everybody's learning process is different, and besides, details in Taiji are just as important as flow. If you don't worry about how large it is or exactly when to turn, you won't really be learning Taiji, which has specific parameters and is not "everything with total freedom." Taiji is a set of specific physical practices that have to be performed with proper regard for the principles and rules of the art, no matter which form you practice. That is not only the definition of form practice, but also part of the discipline. But of course, Huang seems to think that no discipline is necessary. Just step smoothly and wave your arms around in the air in slow motion, and voila, you're doing Taiji. In my experience, it is impossible to practice Taiji unless you are actually practicing Taiji, not empty movements filled with wishful thinking. And finally, it seems to me far better to follow a teacher's instructions than to try to make uo something on my own, completely ignoring the centuries of practical experience bound up in forms.

Or take this statement:

> I have a friend who took a film of an old master in Taiwan by the ocean. It's very beautiful. I may be able to do more fancy things—I have certain skills and a strong body—but that old man had a subtlety, with so many more years of practice, that I can't possible match. So right away, there's no comparison. There's no way of saying, "Your way is better than mine." There's no such thing.

Excuse me, but this last doesn't really make sense. If Taiji is about subtlety, and the old master has a subtlety that Huang can't match, then obviously the old master's way is better. I'm no master, but after more than forty years of practice, I believe that my way of Taiji is superior to the Taiji of a complete tyro with only a few lessons under the belt. And further, Huang says he can do more fancy things than the old master, but is he even considering what the old master was capable of before he got old—all those things that he practiced for decades to give him that subtlety?

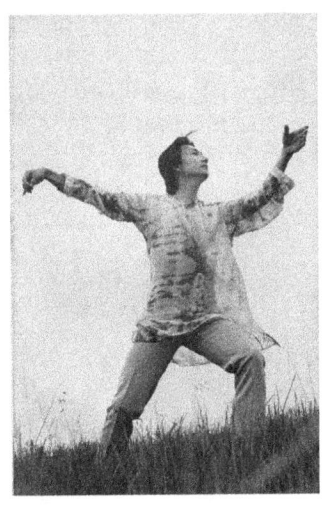

The book is filled with photos, almost all of which are artsy photos of Huang in artsy Taiji poses, sometimes alone, sometimes leading a class. Each of the book's nine chapters is preceded by a full-page photo of Huang in a Taiji pose. I've included one example, but all are very similar. In it, Huang looks relaxed and happy, but what's with the constantly raised chin? It's lifted high in nearly every one of these photos. And sometimes his back is arched inward. Both of these are postural errors that violate basic Taiji principles, which state that the butt and chin should be slightly tucked to open the important acupuncture points in the lower back and back of the neck to allow chi to flow smoothly through the Microcosmic Orbit. Is he so happy because all that chi is flooding into his head with nowhere to go?

Occasionally, though, Huang does manage to make sense.

> T'ai chi needs to be practiced daily in your own movements; it's not something separate that you do only in the morning.

What he's saying is that Taiji isn't isolated from the rest of your life but should, at all times, infuse your movements and spirit with its various effects. So there is wisdom here, but it is so overlaid by a sea of New Age BS that most of the good stuff sinks beneath the waves. In an absolutely perfect world, the New Age stuff might make more sense, but this world is nowhere near perfect and probably never will be. If it were, we wouldn't need Taiji.

Perhaps I am coming to this book with a cup already full, but I see little point in emptying out hard-earned experience for dreck I know to be wrong, no matter who says it. And for me, the form of this book—being a workshop with the author leading through movements—did not work at all. Maybe that approach would suffice for live workshop participants, but it does not in text form, and the result is tedious and only occasionally informative—beyond Huang's free-flowing flow of free-flowing freedom.

There are thousands of Taiji books on the market, and hundreds of good ones, but this isn't one of them. I can't not recommend it enough.

Tai Chi Ch'uan
The Technique of Power

By Tem Horwitz & Susan Kimmelman, with H. H. Lui
(Chicago Review Press, 1976, 234 pages)

Tai Chi Ch'uan: The Technique of Power, by Tem Horwitz and Susan Kimmelman (with H. H. Lui), is a worthwhile addition to Taiji literature. It is not a form-instruction manual; the authors leave that for personal interaction with a live teacher. They write in their preface:

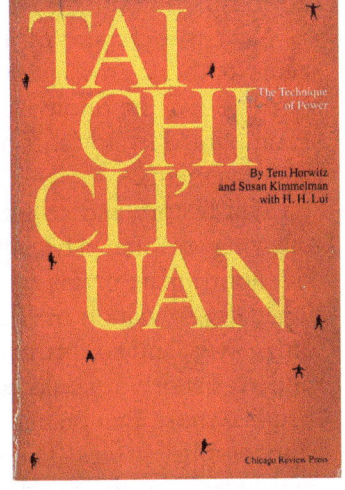

> This book is intended as an introduction and a reference. It is not possible to learn Tai Chi from a book.

Instead, the book is a survey of Taiji, its philosophical background and history, its precepts and methodology, and other Taiji-related matters, such as the Taiji Classics. However, it does have nine pages of small photos of their teacher, H. H. Lui, demonstrating a Taiji form—included, the authors state, merely for reference.

The opening chapter, "Reflections on Getting Up in the Morning," sets the philosophical tone, reminding foremost that existence in reality entails change—change that the authors believe is absolutely necessary for Americans who are trained in efficiency and planned and ordered lives based on rigid social and cultural structures. Taiji and Taoism, they say, are viable methods to help reintroduce meaning and connection into our lives.

The next chapter discusses Taiji in broad terms, laying out its precepts and methodology. It covers the yin/yang dichotomy and defines the meaning and purpose of "form." Throughout, the text is straightforward and refreshingly honest.

Like anything else, in order to get the most out of Taiji, you have to make it your own. In practical terms, this means arranging your life so that you can, and do, practice every day, by yourself. Some teachers claim that ten minutes of daily practice is sufficient. This is false advertising. Taiji is not a magic panacea or any kind of instant short-cut. It's a fair deal—you receive in proportion to what you give.

The authors also council patience because Taiji takes time to mature in the practitioner. This is wisdom that newbies need to heed.

Next is a chapter of H. H. Lui performing a form that largely seems to be a cross between Yang and Wu Family Styles, but as stated above, the photos are meant merely for reference and are not accompanied by any sort of verbal instruction beyond the names of the movements.

Taiji history and an introduction to the Taiji Classics occupy the following chapter. The authors relate the received history of Taiji with appropriate grains of salt, all the way from Bodhidharma to the public dissemination of Taiji by the Chen family and on through the Yangs, Wus, and so forth, marking the beginning of Taiji's established modern history. I would call their take on Taiji history sensible, but they, like most Taiji practitioners, seem to delight in the old, admittedly apocryphal stories. The Classics are not related here, but they are introduced, and their background and importance are discussed. The chapter closes with a limited Taiji family tree.

Readers new to Taiji literature might be thrown a bit by some of the historical names cited by the authors. It's not unusual to see various spellings of names in different Taiji books, but I don't think I've ever seen more unusual ones than here. For example, Wang Tseungyue becomes Wang Chung-yueh, Yang Chengfu becomes Yang Chingpu, Wu Yuxing becomes Woo Yusheong, and Li I-yu is Lee I-yu. Many other names, however, are spelled conventionally, and it's not hard to suss out who the authors are talking about.

The chapter on the Taiji Classics is one of the longest, partly because it takes in not just several of the most important of the standard Taiji Classics, but the *I-Ching* and *Chuang Tzu*, as well.

These passages are ably translated by Lui, and the material is as readable and well-stated as just about any other version of the Classics in Taiji literature and better than many.

The next chapter, "Inner Worlds: Taiji, Mysticism, Magic, Meditation, and Alchemy," delves into these subjects with acceptance that is sensible and practical, but also that is firmly grounded in the nascent New Age philosophies of life and health that were just burgeoning at the time of this book's publication—which also coincided with the first major flowering of Taiji in the United States. Being from that period, it carries some of the excesses of that movement, but not to excess. One passage places this book firmly in its time. On page 172, there is a reference to Carlos Castaneda's *The Teachings of Don Juan: A Yaqui Way of Knowledge*.

I first encountered this book as assigned reading for a course in cultural anthropology in 1969, just after it had been published and when most readers—like the authors of *Tai Chi Ch'uan*—accepted it as a real and true addition to ethnographic literature. This belief took eight sequels and several decades to be thoroughly debunked as fiction, though some readers had been skeptical from the beginning. So it is mildly amusing to see the first in the series cited here as a genuine source to back up claims regarding spirituality. However, most of material the authors present and the sources they cite are much more validly grounded in truth and reality than are Castaneda's works and should be of interest to people with spiritually inquiring minds. (I do have to say, though, that Castaneda's work, fictional though it may be, is not entirely without merit. As the old writerly saw goes, "Sometimes you have to tell a lie to reveal a larger truth.)

The following chapter covers human physical dynamics, exercise, body alignments, kinetics, and chi. Co-author Kimmelman, is a dancer, and a lot of this chapter melds her understanding of human dynamics as well as Taiji. After this comes the final chapter, which continues in a similar vein.

Tai Chi Ch'uan: The Technique of Power is a worthwhile read. Is there anything new here than in other similar books? Not really, but it is better and more deeply stated than in most, and what it says is thorough, encompassing, philosophically moving, and powered by intelligent writing. Recommended primarily for beginners, though intermediate students also would benefit from reading it.

Methods of Applying Taiji Boxing

By Yang Chengfu
(Originally published by the Society for Chinese National Glory, 1931. *Brennan Translations*, 2011, 162 pages)

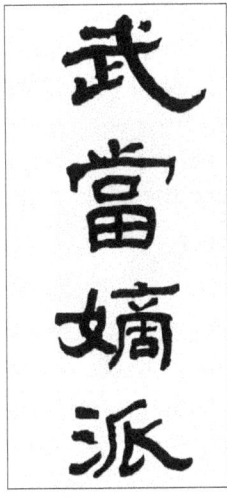

Methods for Applying Taiji Boxing by the historically significant Yang Chengfu has a backstory that might be as interesting as the book. It seems that while Yang was content to teach Taiji to individuals and to display his skill to onlookers, he was initially resistant to disseminating written material on the subject. Despite the fact that the Yang family possessed a number of secret documents on Taiji that most likely included sections of what we now know as the Taiji Classics as well as other material, it all remained closely held within the Yangs' immediate circle.

Until….

According to Stuart Alve Olson, a student of the Yangs named Chen Kung (who later also published under the name Yearning K. Chen and Chen Yanlin), and Chen) obtained permission from Yang Chengfu to take the various notes and transcripts home for one night only to read them. Unknown to Yang, Chen had hired seven transcribers, who copied the manuscripts overnight. Chen returned the materials, but then published the transcripts as his own book. (See Volume VI of this series for reviews of the Chen Kung/Yearning K. Chen/Chen Yanlin books.)

For obvious reasons, this did not sit well with the Yang family, but by then, the cat was out of the bag. In an attempt to reclaim what was theirs, the Yang family subsequently published the material under their own aegis. Hence Yang Chengfu's *Methods of Applying*

Taiji Boxing. As an additional note, it is said that both Chen Weiming and Cheng Man-ching assisted Yang in producing the text, though this also is disputed.

Being ostensibly from the pen of the great Yang Chengfu and containing material not well known at the time of publication, this book was an important Taiji document of its day and still is. Although it contains an extensive instructional section, the more important matters occupy the first twenty and last twelve pages and a dozen pages sandwiched here and there.

Before the text actually begins, Yang leads off with eleven pages that list members of the Yang lineage and prominent students. Many of the names are accompanied by photos, and a great many of these men went on to pen their own books on Taiji.

The first chapter is on the origins of Taiji, and Yang opts for the standard tale of Chang Sanfeng, here called Zhang. Chang witnesses a fight between a bird and a snake in which the snake was victorious thanks to its sinuous flexibility, Taking the hint, Chang then emulated the snake's defense to create Taiji.

Next comes an element that is frequently repeated in the descriptive pages: an anecdote. These anecdotes are about Yang Chengfu's father, Yang Jianhou, his grandfather, Yang Luchan, and his uncle, Yang Banhou. Most of them involve an aggressor attacking one or another of the Yangs, and the stories are not only instructive but interesting and humorous, and they lend human personality to both the text and the art. The first one is about Yang Luchan, but this is Yang Chengfu's book, so you'll have to read it to get the lowdown. You don't see many of these kinds of stories in Taiji books, especially about the great masters, so it's always edifying to read tales about them and their exploits.

A couple of prefaces by students follow that don't add much. Then come "General Remarks," in which Yang delivers pithy statements on the nature and character of Taiji—all basic introductory material for the art. Almost everything here consists of the precepts of Taiji from the Taiji Classics, rewritten and unattributed but valid nonetheless.

Next comes the form instruction section. Or should I say sections since there are several of them with intervening material. First are the instructions for a ninety-four-posture Yang Style consisting of text and a full array of photos of Yang Cheng-fu performing the set. Many of these photos have been reproduced elsewhere, but usually in an abbreviated form and only rarely completely. Unfortunately, the quality of the reproduction is poor.

Push Hands is the next instructional section, and Yang's opponent in the shots is Chen Weiming. The section after contains Taiji Classics by Wang Tsungyueh, here called Wang Zongyue. Each is given in its original before being fully explicated. This sort of dissection of the Classics by authentic experts is de rigueur reading for any Taiji practitioner, and this one is as good as or better than most.

More excerpts from the Taiji Classics follow, including another by Wang Tsungyueh, and that is followed by another instruction section, this one on applications. Then come more Taiji Classics and their explanations.

After that, Yang moves into more-original territory by discussing how to assess and deal with opponents. A discussion of the Eight Gates and Five Steps (the Thirteen Postures/Dynamics) follows. This includes mentions of the Five Elements. Then Yang enumerates several important points to either follow (sticking, adhering, connecting, following) or avoid (crashing in, shallowness, running away, resistance).

Fighting without mistakes and maintaining central ground in fighting are discussed next, and then Yang moves into body posture and Taiji's circling and how they work together. He then gives a mini-treatise on the separation of the civil and martial into three accomplishment in Taiji. Lightness and heaviness, the fundamentals of blood and energy, and refinement of movement are covered next.

There follows an instructional section that has to be one of the most unique in Taiji literature—at least, I've yet to see another example to match it. This is instruction in a two-person Taiji spear set that engages in mock combat to hone skills. One of those anecdotes I mentioned is attached here—this one about Yang Jianhou's skill with the spear.

The final chapter, "Miscellanea," consists of a hodgepodge of disconnected statements on Taiji, some instructional in nature, others merely delivering basic information or another anecdote.

If the story about Chen Kung's appropriation of the Yang family manuscripts is true, and Yang Cheng-fu then scrambled to put out his own book, I would expect the results to look very much like this: a somewhat disconnected mess of really good material. To my mind, the material is poorly organized, jumping back and forth from subject to subject without regard to continuity. I guess mastery of the continuity of movement in Taiji does not necessarily translate into continuity regarding a written work of this scope.

And scope it has, despite its disorganized nature, covering just about every aspect of Taiji, even if if the material is occasionally sketchy or slight. But mostly it's not, delivering excellent information is a fairly readable form. I do wish Yang had been more attentive to his attributions of the Taiji Classics, but he wasn't, so readers just have to understand that he did not originate these ideas.

Considering the provenance of this book, it probably should be read by every serious student of Taiji, no matter what style. Recommended.

T'ai Chi Ch'uan Ta Wen
Questions and Answers on T'ai Chi Ch'uan

by Chen Weiming
Translated by Benjamin Pang Jeng Lo and Robert W. Smith
(North Atlantic Books, 1985, 62 pages)

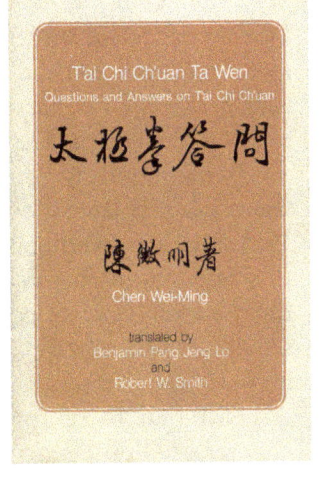

Chen WeiMing's *T'ai Chi Ch'uan Ta Wen* was originally published in 1929. As part of the Chinese Republican Era revival of the martial arts, it is what might be termed a neo-classic. Such books fall between the established Taiji Classics, which were written prior to about 1920, and modern Taiji literature, which began in the 1950s with the initial worldwide diaspora of the art. Chen was one of Yang Chengfu's top student and later established his own schools in Shanghai and elsewhere.

The book principally consists of more than eighty questions asked by Chen during his tutelage, with the answers given by Yang. It's clear, however, that some of the answers are not verbatim responses from Yang but were filtered through Chen since at least once he refers to himself in the first person in an answer. That's not a big deal, per se, since we can assume that Chen didn't have a tape recorder running during his lessons or that he was busily transcribing instead of practicing or listening.

The Q&A comes after a brief preface by translator Benjamin Pang Jeng Lo and an introduction by the author and is broken into a number of category-based chapters:

1) Taichi: Commentary on the History and the Correction of the Legend
2) Taichi: Form
3) Taichi: Push Hands
4) Taichi Fighting Techniques (San Shou)
5) Chin (Jin, Internal Force) of Taichi
6) Relation of Taichi to Tao-yin and Meditation
7) Taichi: Physique and Achievement

Following the Q&A is an appendix containing the Taiji Classic, *Five Character Secret*, by Li I-yu. This material, repeated verbatim from Lo's *The Essence of T'ai Chi Ch'uan: The Literary Tradition*, published six years earlier, seems like so much padding to flesh out a very slender book. If the book were any narrower, there wouldn't be enough room on the spine for the title and author. A five-page glossary closes out the book. There is some good stuff in the glossary, but it is, after all, a glossary, and it's no better than similar glossaries in dozens of Taiji books.

Benjamin Pang Jeng Lo acquired a Chinese language copy of the book and later mentioned it to noted martial arts writer Robert W. Smith, and eventually the two of them undertook the translation that appears in this version. It's difficult to imagine that either of these two important contributors to Taiji and martial arts literature would make a misstep, but this book is not nearly as informative as it could have been considering its sources.

Not that there isn't some good material in these pages. The chapter on Taiji history should not be taken without a grain of salt, but it provides a nice snapshot of Yang Chengfu's beliefs on the subject. And other of the Q&A exchanges are especially good, such as this one, quoted in full:

> Q: Taichi seeks the supple but of what use is suppleness?
> A: Seeking suppleness enables you to separate your body into pieces. If an opponent pushes against your forearm, your elbow doesn't move; if against your shoulder, it moves but not your body; if against your body, it moves but not your waist; if against your waist, it moves but not your leg. This process leaves you as stable as a mountain. When you discharge your opponent, then it is from the feet

through the legs to the waist, body, shoulders, elbows, and hands—all connected as one unit, discharging energy like an arrow toward its target. If you cannot relax, your whole body becomes one piece and, even though it is strong, a stronger person will be able to push your one piece and cause you to be unstable. Thus the use of suppleness is crucial. With it you can be one unit attacking and fragmented parts defending—able to be relaxed and hard, agile stepping forward or back, and substantial and insubstantial as needed. With these abilities you will then have all of the Taichi function.

Unfortunately, the answers to the questions all too often simply refer to the Taiji Classics rather than provide a direct response, and frequently, the responses are as cryptic as anything in the Classics. For example:

Q: When sticking to an opponent what technique can you use to push him while making only a small movement yourself?

A: The Classics contain words which answer this: "If there is up, there is down; if there is forward, there is backward; and if there is left, then there is right." This means to tempt him then attack.

This answer doesn't really address the subject of the question. And some of the questions are the kinds that most people preface with: "I hate to ask a dumb question, but...." For example, Chen asks:

In Taichi postures like Brush Knee, you circle your hand back to the front slowly and then push forward. This is so slow: how could it be functional in a fight?

Yang's answer, though more wordy than this, is that, in a fight, you use appropriate fighting speed. "Otherwise you are being stupid," he concludes, so maybe even he thought it was a dumb question.

And it's not the only one. "Should a novice use force in push-hands?" Chen asks. Anybody with even a smattering of Taiji training should know the answer to this even if they cannot accomplish it on a physical level. "No," Yang responds, but his full answer, which extends into the next question and answer, does provide insight into the proper functioning of the art:

> Be conscientious in Wardoff, Rollback, Press, and Push....These four movements contain limitless change....If he finds your center, change direction quickly but don't disconnect. If your opponent disconnects, quickly push him out.

Some of the exchanges just leave you hanging, wanting more information, such as this one:

> Q: In the fictional work *Chiang Hu Ch'i Hsia Chuan* by Po Hsiao-shen, he criticized the Yang Family and also included a story of Yang Pan-hao. Is this a true account?
> A: This is mere fiction on the level of bickering in the street and cannot be used as evidence. Since scholars are given to jealousy and disputation, how can martial artists who are less educated be free of this fault? There are even gossip and rumors about those with high reputations.

Maybe the author and his contemporaries were in the know about this gossip about Yang Panhou, but the vast majority of readers of this book are not. It seems like a pointless titillation to give a question and answer like this without context. If text fails to give answers or masks information behind reticence, it's best to either add a footnote or leave it out entirely.

And maybe that's the problem with this book. If this was the only such example, I might let it slide. But numerous other examples are scattered throughout the pages, giving the impression of a lot of dross. I guess, though, that if the translators removed all the material that was obvious, foolish, overly cryptic, or repetitive, there wouldn't be a book, only a pamphlet.

While this book might hold some historical interest, it is, at the same time, relatively weak on information, which makes it somewhat disappointing considering its genesis. It has some interesting and useful material but also an equal amount of padding. It probably was more useful in the decades of Republican Era, but there is nothing in here that isn't covered as well or better by the Taiji Classics themselves—or more explicitly and thoroughly by modern Taiji literature.

I'll close with an interesting sidelight. My martial arts library contains one book that I can't read at all since, except for the name of the publisher on the back cover: Hoi Fung Publisher Co. Nor is there is there a date I can read. All the rest—cover and text—is in Chinese. But a look inside is intriguing. After several pages of introductory ideograms, there are portraits on separate pages of Yang Chien-hou, Yang Cheng-fu, and Chen Wei-ming. This is the same portrait of Chen that appears in *T'ai Chi Ch'uan Ta Wen*, and I'm assuming that Chen is the author of this book, too, so that's why I'm including it here.

In his introduction to *T'ai Chi Ch'uan Ta Wen*, Benjamin Lo says that the Chinese edition of the book contained a number of photos of the form that were eliminated in the Lo/Smith translation. The Chinese book under consideration contains a great number of old photos. Following the three portraits just mentioned are seven group photos, presumably of Yang masters and students from various years, and several possibly are of Chen's own schools. From about twenty to about a hundred people are depicted in each photo, and Yang Cheng-fu and other Yang Style notables—including Chen, who is in almost every shot—can be recognized.

However, I don't think that this is the same book because this one appears to then go into a form instruction section instead of a Q&A. The form instruction primarily uses a large number of photos of a young Yang Chengfu, with occasional shots of Chen and a couple of others. After this comes a chapter on push hands with photos depicting a young Yang Chengfu pushing with Chen and another fellow and shots depicting Chen pushing with a man with a beard who looks suspiciously like a young Cheng Man-ching. If so, these photos should put to rest the erroneous assumption that Cheng was not Yang's student. (For more on this controversy, see the review of Robert W. Smith's *Martial Musings: A Portrayal of Martial Arts in the 20th Century*, reviewed in Volume III of this series.) The book winds up with a sequence of photos of the Yang form featuring Chen, though the sequence is not complete, truncating before the last few movements.

Chen wrote several books on Taiji and related subjects, but I don't have a comprehensive list of his titles (that I can read), so I might never know which one this is. But even so, I value this book for its many historic photos.

See the next review for an alternate translation of *T'ai Chi Ch'uan Ta Wen*.

Answering Questions about Taiji
Including Single Posture Practice Methods

By Chen Weiming
(Originally published 1929. *Brennan Translations*, 2012, 88 pages)

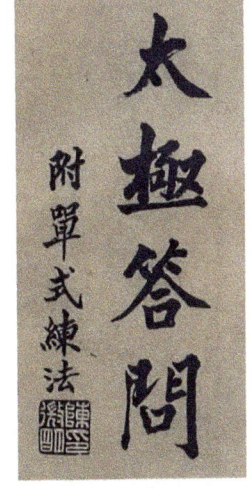

This book is an alternate translation of Chen Weiming's *T'ai Chi Ch'uan Ta Wen*—a transcribed Q&A regarding the art of Taiji. This particular version is more complete than the one translated by Benjamin Pang Jeng Lo and Robert W. Smith, reviewed just above.

Except for the exact verbiage used, the two books cover the same material for the first seven chapters. The translations of the chapters that appear in both books may not be identical, but there is little difference between them aside from exact verbiage. so I'll let the previous review do double-duty in describing that material.

However, there are some significant differences. From the chart on the next page, you can see that the Brennan translation contains several chapters that don't appear in the Lo/Smith translation. Only the first two of these are actually germane to the contents of the book. The others are on aspects of the Achieving. Softness Boxing Society, which Chen founded in about 1924. The Lo/Smith book has its own preface and introduction, while the Brennan translation contains Chen's original preface.

The first of the extra chapters, "On Taiji Boxing's Benefits," continues the Q&A with two issues: "Does Taiji Have Any Proven Effects on the Body?" and "Should Women Practice Taiji Boxing?" Chen answers both with a resounding, "Yes" and some more verbiage to back him up. The second extra chapter contains a twenty-four posture Yang Style form with textual instructions and some-

Lo / Smith	Brennan
1) Preface (by Benjamin Pang Jeng Lo)	1) Preface (by Chen Weiming)
2) Introduction	2) None
3) Taiji: Commentary on the History and the Correction of the Legend	3) On Embellishments to Taiji Boxing's Origins and Pointing Out Falsehoods within Fiction
4) Taiji Form	4) On Taiji Boxing's Postures
5) Taiji Push Hands	5) On Taiji Boxing's Pushing Hands
6) Taiji Fighting Techniques (San Shou)	6) On Taiji Boxing's Various Techniques
7) Chin (Internal Force) of Taiji	7) On Taiji Boxing's Energies
8) Relation of Taiji to Tao-yin and Meditation	8) On Taiji Boxing's Methods of Limbering and Meditation
9) Taiji: Physique and Achievement	9) The Taiji Student's Build versus Accomplishment
10) None	10) On Taiji Boxing's Benefits
11) None	11) On Taiji Boxing's Single-Posture Practice Methods
12) None	12) List of Achieving Softness Boxing Society Members
13) None	13) List of Instructors Teaching Beyond the School
14) None	14) Achieving Softness Boxing Society's General Rules
15) None	15) Achieving Softness Boxing Society's General Rules for Outside Instructors
16) None	16) Achieving Softness Boxing Society's Three-Year Graduate Program
17) Five-Character Secret by Li I-yu	17) None
18) Glossary	18) None

what mediocre photos of Chen doing the demonstrating. The chapters on the Achieving Softness Boxing Society finish the book with a bunch of material that would be of interest and value only to historians of the martial arts.

In comparing the two translations of this book, I have to come down on the side of Brennan's effort, if only because it has those extra chapters. Its translation is just as cogent, seems a little more thorough, and contains Chen's original introduction. Plus, it's free.

Cheng Tzu's Thirteen Treatises on T'ai Chi Ch'uan

by Cheng Man-ch'ing
Translated by Benjamin Pang Jeng Lo & Martin Inn
(North Atlantic Books, 1985, 224 pages)

Master Cheng's Thirteen Chapters on T'ai-Chi Ch'üan

by Cheng Man-ch'ing
translated by Douglas Wile
(Sweet Ch'i Press, 1982, 72 pages)

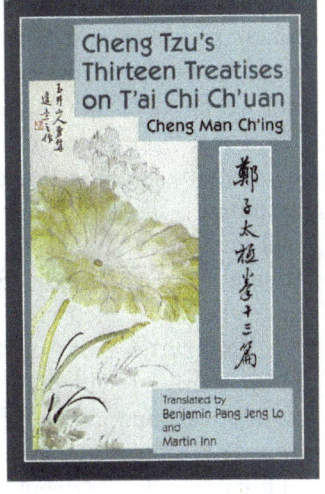

Cheng Man-ch'ing is justly revered as a primary disseminator of Taijiquan in America. His expertise attracted a number of students who went on to become members of America's first wave of homegrown masters and who continue to broadcast Cheng's 37-posture Yang Style across the United States and the world. His writings on the art —some written for the English-speaking audience, some translated from earlier works in Chinese—are among the earlier books on Taiji in English, though they are by no means the earliest thanks to belatedly late translations.

Cheng studied Taiji with Yang Cheng-fu for the last six years of Yang's life and reportedly helped ghostwrite Yang's second book on Taiji: *Essence and Applications of Tai Chiquan* (alternately titled, *The Substance and Application of T'ai Chi Ch'uan*), which was published in 1934. In the thirteenth chapter of the *Thirteen Chapters*, Cheng expresses trepidation about publishing a book that reveals Taiji's secrets, and that Yang Cheng-fu was equally reluctant to write about Taiji for fear of exposing the art to those who might misuse it. However, in 1925, one of Yang's students, *Chen Weiming*, published *The Art of T'ai-chi Ch'üan*, and not long after, another student, Chen Kung (aka. Chen Yanlin, Yearning K. Chen), published his own book based on materials purloined from Yang, so Yang finally relented, enlisting Cheng to assist him in writing his own book. (See Volume VI of this series for reviews of Chen Kung's books.)

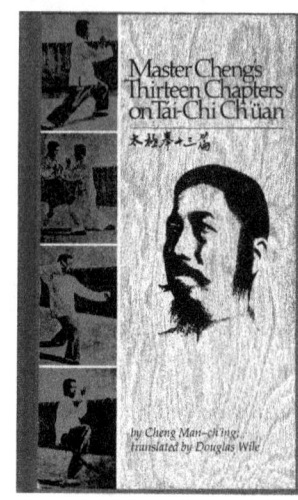

Subsequent to Yang's death in 1936, Cheng penned *Thirteen Chapters*, which was completed in 1947 but not published until 1950, making this the first book published under his own name. In essence, Cheng's *Thirteen Chapters*—along with the books of his near contemporaries, Chen Weiming and Chen Kung—can collectively be considered as sturdy primary struts of a bridge between the older works on Taiji, known as the Taiji Classics, and modern Taiji literature.

To my knowledge, *Thirteen Chapters* has been translated into English twice, and I'm going to review both books here because, essentially, it's the *Thirteen Chapters* that is important. And this also will give me a chance to go over the primary material—Cheng's information—separately from the secondary material—the differences between the two books.

Thirteen Chapters seems to me to be a prototypical nuts-'n-bolts book, many of which combine history, philosophy, and precepts with in-depth examinations of dynamics, energy movement, and purpose. Some of these sorts of books also contain form instruction material, in greater or lesser detail, and personal insights or anecdotes.

Thirteen Chapters can be difficult to read, but not because the language is deliberately abstruse or because the subject matter can't be comprehended. For the most part, Cheng imparts his information clearly and in great enough detail to make it useful. The book's difficulty lies in the fair share of serious weaknesses that mar its many strengths. There is, for example, a passage where Cheng diverges into lengthy discussions on cultivating and amassing chi that are not as well explicated as some of the other material and that often can seem like magical thinking. If chi is a tangible force, then we should have a more tangible theory about its creation, storage, movement, and so forth. But I do have to agree with his overall assessment that Taiji is a form of personal alchemy.

And some of Cheng's other arguments are marred by statements or notions that seem to be nonsense by today's standards, such as his claim that swimming can cause gonorrhea. Or this:

> Our solar system may be considered so great that nothing can contain it....If its form were not circular, then in spite of the power of accumulated ch'i, it could not be supported and could not float the countless stars in space, all in revolution.

Okay, maybe I'm nit-picking here, but his physics and cosmology need a little work.

The idea does make better sense, though, if you substitute "The universe" for "Our solar system." But it is true—unfortunately for his argument—that while some galaxies revolve, others, such nebulae and elliptical and shell galaxies, do not. And there are many large star clusters that seem to hold together despite their lack of rotation. And on the incredibly macro scale, there are huge gaps and voids around which galactic clusters, swarm like soap froth around emptiness, none of which is necessarily revolving. My complaints here have a purpose. If you are going to use science to help explain something, make sure the science is at least reasonably accurate, otherwise, errors stand out disproportionally. Just like in push hands.

When it comes to Cheng's discussions of Taiji dynamics, however, his analogies are more apt and illustrative and are very welcome. He begins with the concept of "roundness," including the ideas of central stability and centrifugal and centripetal forces, and the complementary concepts of squareness and triangulation. From there, he delves into the absorption and release of energy, leverage, and uprooting. There are lots of diagrams in this chapter to help illustrate the concepts.

Cheng was noted for his medical knowledge, but reading through the chapter on the health benefits of Taiji make me glad it's seventy years later and that he's not my doctor. I don't want to disparage traditional Chinese medicine, but I am always leery when someone claims that Taiji can cure cancer, tuberculosis, or other severe and frequently fatal diseases. In relation to the lungs, Cheng writes:

> They…cannot be directly reached by Western medicine's needles or drugs. Apart from surgery or inner cultivation, I have never heard of any effective cures for lung disorders. (Wile, p. 42)

Perhaps there were fewer such treatments when Cheng wrote this book, but I think that, even at the time, a little research on the topic would have showed him that this statement is incorrect. There are, in fact, drugs and needles that can reach formerly inaccessible places and perform formerly impossible tasks—take the Epipen, for example. He even contradicts himself just a few pages later when he tells of curing many cases of tuberculosis, or seeing patients cured, by various means, including eating ducks force-fed on human placenta, boar's lungs into which the juice of twelve uncooked chickens have been poured, and large doses of cinnamon, ginseng, and other herbs. I guess all that can be considered "drugs" since they are take for medicinal reasons. Pardon me, but I think I'll stick to antibiotics. Also untrue is the statement:

> Lung disease can only be resisted through spirit and courage, otherwise there will be rapid deterioration. (Wile, p. 42)

Good spirits, courage, and effort certainly are necessary in combatting any illness or injury, but good medical treatment—whether Eastern or Western—is pretty vital, too. And heck, now we can treat some lung diseases with drugs or palliatives, remove diseased lung tissue, and even transplant whole lungs.

Don't get me wrong: I'm not disparaging either Western or traditional Chinese medicine. From what I can tell, they both work pretty well within their spheres and probably would work best if they worked together. Nor is it to say that I don't believe that chi-building exercises help affect a positive outcome. I do. Taiji and chi kung can aid almost any condition by daily bathing all the tissues in the body with extra-strong doses of chi's healing vitality. And chi kung can further direct and focus that healing energy into specific tissue where it's needed. But it is in the maintenance of daily health that Taiji and chi kung excel, and when it comes to illness or injury, other measures usually are necessary as well.

In discussing the escalating stages of development within the Taiji exponent, Cheng offers more solid advice than he does in the chapter on medicine. This chapter discusses how the chuanist learns to sense and then control the various bodily connections that, when added together, impart coordinated, whole-body movement and power. It's a good prescription—and good advice—and elucidated well enough to follow and benefit from.

Cheng then goes into a section on the yin and yang of energy embodied in the Taiji form. In this, he relies almost exclusively on the idea of the sequence of creation and destruction of forces expounded in the theory of the Five Elements. This is all well and good, but I'd rather see something that relies a little more on mechanics than on abstract theory. Metal defeats wood...okay, let's see, now, which moves are metal and which are wood? Maybe I'll get it eventually, if I ever have the time....

The book winds up with a chapter containing twelve statements from Yang Chengfu, complete with paragraphs by Cheng interpreting the meanings of those statements. Most of us have read Yang's words before and seen them interpreted, but who better to repeat and interpret them than Cheng since the words of both these masters carry import even on multiple readings.

I know I've been hard on this book at times, but that is only because it is a landmark work, and landmark works invite scrutiny. Nor should a reviewer overlook inconsistencies, weaknesses, or outright nonsense if they are noticed, no matter how knowledgeable or impressive the author might be. Over all, I have to say that this book is poised in a 70/30 stance: 70 percent solid and 30 percent empty.

Now, let's compare the two versions. The titles of the two delineate the primary difference between the two books. Douglas Wile titles his, *Master Cheng's Thirteen Chapters on T'ai-Chi Ch'üan*, while Benjamin Pang Jeng Lo and Martin Inn title theirs, *Cheng Tzu's Thirteen Treatises on T'ai Chi Ch'uan*. You say "potAto," I say, "poTAHto." Obviously differences in the tenor of the language of the translations exist between the two. How could that not be? But without personally undertaking translation from Chinese to English or going to the trouble to parse the two versions side-by-side to determine which verbiage one likes best, it would be difficult to tell which one to buy. Translation is an art of its own. Note, for example, the following two passages, which illustrate how the language of a translation can punch up the meaning. Cheng is talking about soft vs hard:

> We may compare this with the teeth, which are firm and hard, and the tongue, which is soft. Occasionally, the teeth and tongue have disagreements and the tongue must temporarily invest in loss.... (Wile, p.1)

> For example, the teeth are hard and the tongue is soft. When the teeth and tongue do not properly meet, the tongue will be temporarily useless.... (Lo/Inn, p. 22)

In this sentence, Wile is clearly more on the ball, employing double entendre gleaned from Taiji precepts—keep your teeth lightly closed to prevent biting your tongue—in addition to using good comic timing. Lo/Inn's, on the other hand, seems a bit awkward, and its meaning is unclear—exactly how is the tongue useless if it and the teeth don't meet properly? My tongue and teeth meet all sorts of ways, but my tongue only becomes useless when I bite it or when I'm too dumbfounded to speak. Presumably Lo means that the teeth should meet lightly, with the tip of the tongue touching the hard palate, but that's not what he says.

I don't intend to imply here that the Wile translation is superior to the Lo/Inn. I'm simply using this one example to show how the particular wording of a translation can heighten meaning or lend some appropriate humor or drama. There are many instances where the Lo/Inn translation is more subtle or to the point than the Wile. Also to be fair, the Lo/Inn version came out a couple of years after Wile's, so they had to take the trouble not only to translate, but to ensure they didn't translate it exactly as Wile had.

So, really, in choosing between the books—if you must—the quality of the translations isn't the issue. Some might prefer the Lo/Inn version simply because it contains more material than the Wile. Here is a breakdown of the material in each:

Lo / Inn
(224 pages)
Introduction by Madam Cheng
Introduction by Benjamin Pang-jeng Lo
Bio of Cheng Man-ching by Min Hsiaochi
The Thirteen Chapters
Explanation of the Essential Points
Professor Yang's Essential Points of T'ai Chi Ch'uan
The Respected Transmission
Form Instruction
Push Hands
Q&A
"Song of Substance and Function"
Glossary

Wile
(72 pages)
Translator's Note
Bio of Cheng Man-ching by Min Hsiaochi
Author's Preface (Cheng)
The Thirteen Chapters

Wile's is the no-frills model—Cheng's *Thirteen Chapters* with its original introduction—while Lo and Inn's contains enough additional material to triple Wile's page count. In both versions, the *Thirteen Chapters* itself occupies roughly the same number of pages: seventy-two in Wile, seventy-seven in Lo/Inn (which utilizes a larger font and looser leading). But for those who own Cheng's *T'ai-Chi: The "Supreme Ultimate" Exercise for Health, Sport, and Self-Defense* (See review in Volume VI of this series), the form instruction and push hands sections, which take up the lion's share of the additional pages in the Lo/Inn version, are superfluous and actually inferior to the material contained the other book.

What remains is a smattering of useful information in the three very brief chapters coming immediately after the *Thirteen Chapters*, in the Q&A, in the one Taiji Classic ("Song of Substance and Function"), and in the "Glossary." The latter contains many good and clearly stated concepts that are valuable, even for those with some experience at Taiji. But of course, we have Lo and Inn to thank for that, rather than Cheng. Then there is the introduction by Madam Cheng, which lends heart to the book. And finally, the cover art is a painting by Cheng himself. Most Taijiquanists don't realize it, but Cheng's art is what initially brought him to America, not Taiji.

Clearly, I own both books, so I never made the choice between the two. I guess I believe that slightly different perspectives on the same material can't be a bad thing. After all, two people can learn Taiji from the same teacher and exhibit differences in their forms—differences that aren't necessarily right or wrong but are just different. Furthermore, different expressions of the same source material can be instructive.

To me, the *Thirteen Chapters* is what's important. Cheng was a powerful presence in the Taiji community: a bridge-builder not just between between classic and modern Taiji but between mastery of Taiji in China and mastery of it in the United States. He was personally responsible for training a core of American Taiji players, many who became well known for their expertise and who have further developed the art and passed it on to new generations of students. Moreover, the *Thirteen Chapters*—in either translation—is the first of Cheng's two most substantially stated works on Taiji and is a significant addition to Taiji literature. If the work contains some stuff that's less than optimal, so be it. Deflect the bad and receive the good.

Sources

"Cheng Man-ching." *Wikipedia*, https://en.wikipedia.org/wiki/Cheng_Man-ch%27ing

"Chen Weiming." *Wikipedia*, https://en.wikipedia.org/wiki/Chen_Weiming_(scholar)

The Tai Chi Book
Refining and Enjoying a Lifetime of Practice

by Robert Chuckrow
(YMAA Publication Center, 1998, 210 pages)

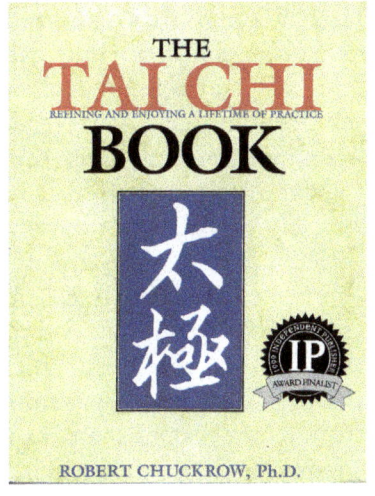

Robert Chuckrow is the author of, as far as I can tell, four books on Taiji. *The Tai Chi Book* is, apparently, the second of these. I have a reason for saying "apparently." His first book, released in 1995, was titled *T'ai chi ch'uan: Embracing the Pearl: Including the Teachings of Cheng Man-ch'ing, William C.C. Chen, and Harvey I. Sober*, and the sub-sub title to *The Tai Chi Book* is *Including the Teachings of Cheng Man-ch'ing, William C.C. Chen, and Harvey I. Sober*. So it's unclear to me if *The Tai Chi Book* is an expansion of the earlier work, or if both just happen to include teachings from the Taiji experts named in both subtitles, all of whom Chuckrow learned from. I'd buy the earlier book to find out, but it is out of print and used copies go for $150, so for now, I'll just have to invest in loss and accept my ignorance.

The Tai Chi Book is a very good manual intended for the beginner and intermediate student. In it, Chuckrow delves into various aspects of Taiji with, as can be guessed by the three experts named in the sub-sub title, an emphasis on the style developed by Cheng Man-ch'ing (Zheng Manquing). With a Ph.D. in physics, the author brings to bear a scientific approach to understanding the dynamics of Taiji, and with a background in teaching both physics and Taiji, he knows how to present his material well.

He opens the book with a few brief remarks before getting into the first chapter: "What is T'ai Chi Ch'uan?" The chapter begins with his discovery of Taiji—fortuitously that taught by Cheng Man-ch'ing, perhaps the art's leading exponent in the United States at that time. He then delineates several aspects of what Taiji "is": a spiritual teaching, a form of meditation, a system of health and healing, a physical expression of Taoist philosophy, and a system of self-defense. He spends several to many pages on each of these subjects, delving into some of the deeper aspects of each.

Chapter two is titled, simply, "Ch'i." Elements he discusses here are chi kung, what chi is in broad terms, the benefits of strengthening one's chi, how chi is experienced, a possible scientific basis for chi, why some people fail to experience chi, sensing and cultivating chi, sending chi, the effects of clothing on chi, chi possessed by inanimate objects, feng shui (geomancy), cautions about chi, and why the existence of chi is hard for some people to accept.

The next chapter covers a number of basic ideas, concepts and principles of Taiji. Early on, he quotes Cheng Man-ch'ing, who was master of the Five Excellences: painting, traditional Chinese medicine, Taiji, calligraphy, and poetry. When Cheng was asked which of the five was the most difficult, he replied, "T'ai Chi Ch'uan is the hardest because it has more principles than any of the others." Chuckrow expands on this, writing, "Not only are the principles numerous, but they require consistent practice over an extended period of time."

He then proceeds to describe these principles in brief or longer subsections: air, balance, centering, chi, circles, concentration, continuity, double weighting, drawing silk (silk reeling), gravity, levelness of motion, leverage, macroscopic and microscopic movement, Newton's First Law (which defines the inertia of motion and rest), Newton's Third Law (which states that a force generates an equal and opposite force), opening and closing of the joints, peng, perpetual motion, precision, rotation, sensitivity, separation of yin and yang, sequence of motion, shape, spatial relationships, stepping, sticking, strength, sung (sinking/relaxation), suspension of the head, unity of movement, the body's axis, vision, and visualization.

If you think that's a run-on sentence, then just consider it to be a long form, flowing like a river.

Breathing is the subject of chapter four. The author begins with everyday breathing and efficient or inefficient breathing. He then moves on to Taiji breathing, or more properly, abdominal breathing. Chapter five looks at body alignments, beginning with a definition of alignment and reasons why awareness of alignment is important, before moving on to discuss obstacles to proper alignment. Chuckrow then provides details regarding the alignments of specific joints and linked joint groups in the arms, the legs, the torso, and the neck and head. Warm-ups and stretching are examined in the following chapter. The importance of flexibility are looked at first, followed by a number of important concepts about stretching.

Chapter seven takes on stances, which are the foundation of Taiji's solidity and its ability to dissipate and expel energy. Here, Chuckrow introduces a number of terms linked with particular stances, such as parallel stance, empty stance, and double weighting. These concepts find further explication in descriptions of several key Taiji stances, such as 50/50, 70/30, and 100/0 percent. He also helpfully includes warnings about how certain faulty alignments not only adversely affect stances and their stability, but can inadvertently lead to injury.

The next chapter, "On Being a Student," leads off with what has to be the most important idea in all of Taiji: a commitment to dedicated practice over a long period of time. He also discusses group vs individual practice, the length of practice sessions, practicing indoors vs outdoors, time of day to practice, self-discipline, how to deal with the fear of making mistakes, one's mental state during practice, varying practice speed, mirror image practice (see below), practice in different locations, and several other aspects. He includes here some exercises for improving balance. He then goes into teachers of Taiji, from choosing a teacher to teaching methods, and how one should assess teachers. He finishes with a number of pages of advice to beginners, from understanding the learning process to measuring progress. Learning from books and videos also is covered here.

Health, healing, and sexuality are the subjects of chapter nine. He begins with several pages on injuries, learning from injuries, and treating various types of basic injuries such as bruises, sprains, tendonitis, and cuts. A section on massage follows, and after that, the author moves down to the feet, which often are neglected but which are the only true foundation for the body. Brief discussions of nutrition, sexuality, and sleep round out the chapter.

Chapter ten covers a number of miscellaneous matters, such as art and Taiji, science and Taiji, and comparisons of long and short forms. Variations in the forms of great masters, such as how much the rear leg is bent and using a straight or bent wrist, are examined next.

The final chapter takes on push hands, from basic one-handed forms through moving two-handed forms. Here, again, principles dominate, such as yielding, neutralization, correct force, rooting, receiving energy, sticking, listening, and non-action, among many others. The book closes with an appendix showing Chuckrow demonstrating Cheng Man-ch'ing's thirty-seven posture short form.

While this is, to all extents and purposes, a book for the beginner and intermediate student—and it covers all the bases for students at those levels—it is unusual in including a great deal more information on health and well-being than do most such books.

A lot of the material the author covers could be dry and uninterestingly stated, but Chuckrow is too good a writer and teacher for that. He continually livens things up with anecdotes and personal stories to give life to the concepts he writes about. This makes the book more interesting as well as sinking in the points he makes.

I do have to comment on one element mentioned above. Early on, Chuckrow states that Cheng Man-ch'ing taught that one should not perform Taiji in left-handed, or, mirror-image forms. Cheng's reasoning was that the two sides of the body are not symmetrical with regards to the placement of internal organs and that, while the energies generated by doing the usual, right-handed form are beneficial, they can be detrimental when generated by doing the form in mirror image.

I was taught nearly four decades ago to do the form on both sides to help balance the body, and I don't appear to have suffered any adverse effects. Further, I've seen that doing the form in mirror image actually expands its martial repertoire. Some of the applications in the right-handed form can only deal with left-handed attacks, which are less likely than right-handed attacks, and doing the form on both sides enables the practitioner to utilize the full range of applications on either side. Chuckrow doesn't go into this idea, in particular, though later in the book, he does discuss doing the form in mirror image in more positive terms.

Another thing I like about the book is that the author places the footnotes for each chapter at the end of the chapter instead of at the end of the book, making it easy for readers to flip to learn more if a particular footnote strikes a chord of interest.

One final note: *The Tai Chi Book* was a 1999 Independent Publishers Award Finalist.

While there are a number of excellent Taiji books for the beginner on the market, this one easily stacks up.

Tai Chi Dynamics
Principles of Natural Movement, Health, and Self-Development

by Robert Chuckrow
(YMMA Publications Center, Inc., 2008, 252 pages)

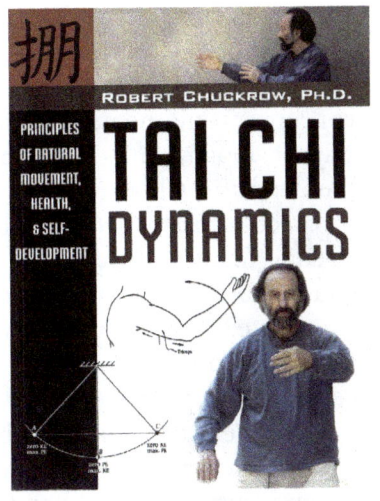

Among books on Taiji, there are the good, bad, and those in the middle ground. Among the good ones, there are those that are pretty good, very good, and really, really good. I'd place Robert Chuckrow's *Tai Chi Dynamics* near the top of the scale. This book occupies a space somewhere between philosophical/scientific works and a nuts-'n-bolts book. It has a fair share of discussion of how Taiji functions on a practical level—which includes energy manipulations as well as physical movement—but it also delves deeply into principles and methodology.

Chuckrow, who has a Ph.D. in experimental physics and taught that subject at a private school for most of his career, studied with Cheng Man-ch'ing, William C. C. Chen, and Harvey I Sober, among others. His Taiji credentials are as solid as his knowledge of physics, and both inform and lend a great deal of credibility to what he has to say.

Chuckrow opens with a chapter titled, "Muscular Action in Taiji Movement," which discusses the need for strength in the martial arts as well as the different kinds of strength possible for one to employ. Taiji's "tenacious strength," jin, is contrasted to muscular strength, or li, following which, Chuckrow writes:

> This chapter attempts to analyze muscular action in a way that should reduce the time for practitioners to understand the distinction between jin and li.

This "attempt" runs through several subsections titled, "Force," "Muscular Action: Contraction and Extension," "A Reconsideration of Zheng's [Cheng Man-ch'ing] Distinction Between the Two Types of Strength," "Implied Strength," "Peng," Muscular Action and Yin and Yang," and Sympathetic Muscular Tension."

Throughout, the information is solid and practical, and one of the main takeaways from this excellent parsing of strength and muscular action is the linking of jin with muscular extension rather than muscular contraction. Chuckrow learned the concept of muscular extension from Elaine Summers, and while I'd never heard the concept given a name, I immediately recognized the validity of this way of looking at—and experiencing—Taiji movements. I'll leave the details to Chuckrow, but in short, muscular extension asks you to execute movements by elongating muscles rather than by contracting them. In other words, if you hold your arm out in front of you, palm up, there are two ways you can make your forearm pivot on your elbow to cause your palm to move toward your face. The first is to contract your bicep, and the second is to extend your triceps. Taiji employs the latter.

The next chapter is on breathing and covers natural breathing and reverse breathing and presents a few exercises to help the practitioner engage in diaphragmatic—or, abdominal—breathing. The author spends time on a number of aspects involved in breathing that most Taiji books either gloss over or do not cover at all. This is a shame because proper breathing is essential to generate and propel chi through the meridians, so thanks go to Chuckrow for his insights on this subject.

The chapter that follows, which occupies a little more than twenty pages, is where Chuckrow's science background comes to the fore. Titled, "Relationships of Conditions, Shape, Timing, Muscular Action, and Yin and Yang in Taiji Movements," it is a far-ranging examination of Taiji dynamics that begins by defining relative body motion before defining movement along three principal planes. He includes concepts such as parallax, which he defines as "the apparent relative movement of two objects at different distances from an observer, resulting from movement of the observer." When you're driving down the road, parallax is responsible for the telephone poles next to the road to see to be zipping past while the mountains in the background are barely creeping along. Parallax, Chuckrow writes, "can also be useful in a self-defense situation if properly utilized in conjunction with the myriad other ways of processing information."

He discusses the circularity of Taiji movements next, which includes footwork as well as arm and hand movements. Next he delves into how the body displays both convexity and concavity and how those curvatures, or bows, can be employed to make the body's movements more subtle as well as more powerful. The way that many Taiji movements begin and end with various parts moving simultaneously is discussed next, and this segues naturally into a section on stepping. Muscular extension plays a role here, as do the natural swing of the leg when stepping and the idea of solid/empty stances. Other elements, such as concentration and practicing on rough surfaces finish out the chapter.

"Dynamics of Movement" is the title of the next chapter, which, in thirty pages, delivers more solid information on how Taiji functions than a whole shelf of average Taiji books do. The concepts are almost too numerous to enumerate here, and certainly I'll have to leave it to Chuckrow's own words to add detail. He starts with the idea that movement is either yin or yang, and uses that to explain how movement is affected by, uses, or produces inertia, equal and opposite action and reaction, gravity, leverage, centrifugal force, linear and angular momentum, peng, torque, hydraulic pressure, kinetic energy, potential energy, spring energy, periodic motion, vibration, wave motion, and intention.

This is fascinating reading, containing a great number of excellent concepts that are all well explained. He then goes on to show how Taiji movements can transform one type of mechanical energy into another. Shifting of weight and turning the body correctly wind up this chapter. I really appreciate it when a Taiji author brings a wide range of knowledge to bear on the subject, since, indeed, Taiji finds significant connections and parallels throughout reality.

A chapter titled "Seemingly Paradoxical Admonitions" is next. This consists, in essence, of maxims from the Taiji Classics recast as simple statements that the author then explicates at some length within the framework of Taiji. This is followed by a chapter on stretching, focusing on muscular extension.

Push hands and applications occupy the next two chapters. Most of the chapter on push hands is not specifically practical but is more concerned with motivation, principles, connection between partners, balance, and leverage. Helpful is a list of push-hands errors. The chapter on applications is, in a sense, obligatory, and it's probably the weakest chapter in the book. The dozen or so applications are basic, and while they are adequately discussed in text and two to three photos each, this section isn't any different or better than similar sections in scores of Taiji books. But I suppose the applications do illustrate certain concepts of which beginners might not be aware, even if this book seems geared more for the intermediate and advanced student. The photos are somewhat fuzzy or murky, which tends to be the case with the photography throughout the book, though it's not especially distracting.

A far-ranging look at Taiji as a martial art follows. It includes subsections on modern self-protection tools, chin na, falling and rolling, deception, distancing, laws pertaining to the use of weapons and deadly force, throwing objects, striking, anatomy, grappling, taking punches, hiding and evading, knots, survival in extreme conditions, crime, and creativity in utilizing self-defense. Most of these are very short and don't really contain specific information or advice but serve more as reminders to consider these elements at greater length on one's own.

Cheng Man-ch'ing is the subject of the book's next chapter. It's a short but pithy chapter that drops a lot of names and relates several anecdotes about Cheng, all of which is fun as well as interesting. Of note is a digression on Cheng's teachings on the use of strength and yielding, and how his ideas might have been erroneously fastened on by some practitioners.

The author then devotes a long chapter to health, including the effects of muscular action, external influences, sexual activity, pain, self-massage, and fasting. He includes a list of more than thirty famous Taiji masters, along with the dates of their births and deaths and their life spans in years. One of the promotional words used to advertise tai chi is "longevity," and this chart goes a long way to dispelling the myth that Taiji, alone, will make you live longer. Yang Cheng-fu, for example, was only fifty-three when he died. T.T. Liang, though, reached 102. To my mind, Taiji doesn't necessarily promote longevity in the sense of a longer life, but rather, enables practitioners to move as if they are younger than their actual age.

Self-development occupies the next chapter. This material is primarily philosophical in tone rather than instructional, but there is a lot of practical advice, too. A great deal of the material in this chapter isn't directly related to Taiji, but as Taiji practitioners come to realize, everything about you affects your Taiji, and your Taiji affects everything about you. It becomes easy, after a time, to draw parallels between your Taiji practice and other elements of your life and environment. In subsections like "Laughter," "Negativity," "Regret," and "Criticism," Chuckrow gives the reader a quiet rendition of a prescription for better living, and through that, a way to develop the self in accord with not only what should be, but what is. Included is a Q&A section in which he gives answers to questions about life that he was asked by his physics students.

The chapter after primarily concerns teaching Taiji, from practical suggestions to where to teach, how to teach, how much to charge, how to deal with class administration, and other related matters. This chapter has information useful to beginners seeking a teacher, but it is obviously geared more toward those thinking of teaching Taiji on their own, which isn't an activity for beginners.

A chapter on miscellaneous items winds up the book. It talks about, among other things, the Romanization of Chinese words, sweating, skeletal relationships, persistence, content versus outer appearance, and studying with teachers who interpret Taiji matters differently. Included are instructions for making your own Taiji slippers, complete with a pattern.

Chuckrow has an easy, comfortable style of writing that makes it seem like you're just sitting there, listening to him talk. The pages are seasoned with anecdotes and personal stories that help illustrate his points with examples from a variety of life-learning experiences. But that easy style manages to convey a great deal of complex substance. The book is loaded with diagrams, illustrations, and photos to supplement the text. No Taiji book is perfect, but *Tai Chi Dynamics* is as good as it gets and surveys a lot of important territory.

Taiji Boxing Explained

By Yao Fuchun and Jiang Rongqiao
(Originally published by Shanghai Martial Studies Press, 1930. *Brennan Translations*, May 2016. 318 pages.)

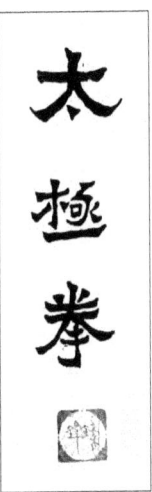

There are a lot of standard-fare Taiji manuals out there, but this isn't one of them. In *Taiji Boxing Explained*, Yao Fuchun and Jiang Rongqiao do a pretty good job of living up to the title of the book.

The book follows the general pattern of most Taiji manuals, both old and new: prefatory material, historical material, and principles and methodology, followed by a form instruction section, information on push hands, and a chapter on the Taiji Classics. What sets this book apart is the quality and quantity of information contained in each of these sections.

For example, *Taiji Boxing Explained* has an astounding seven prefaces—one each by the authors, two by a pair of Jiang's teachers, one by swordsman Li Li, and a couple by Yao's students. Some of the prefatory material is simply introductory, but some of it has meat. To give you an idea of the scope of this hefty book, all this prefatory material plus the table of contents takes up about thirty pages.

The origins of Taiji are shrouded in a non-literate past. By this I mean that the history of its invention and development was not formally recorded, not that the Chinese of the time were necessarily illiterate. So, barring the discovery of definitive historical texts that either no longer exist or never did, we have to take the legendary histories of Chang Sanfeng and his successors as apocryphal at best. But in the Americas and Europe, we are at a disadvantage because mostly we hear the same old stories of Chang's art eventually reaching the Chen family via Wang Tsungyueh or Chiang Fa, or both, among others. After reading a number of older Chinese Taiji manuals translated by Paul Brennan, it has become clear to me that this basic origins story has many permutations and details that have not yet been absorbed by Western practitioners.

The authors of *Taiji Boxing Explained* begin their historical essay on the origins of Taiji with a bio of Chang. The difference between this bio and the fare usually presented in Taiji manuals is that Chang's acquisition of the art is not only mystical but practical, naming Lu Chunyang and Zheng Liulong as masters from whom Chang obtained the Natural Way and the Uppermost Way, respectively. Of course it is impossible to separate the mystical from the art and practice of Taiji, so the authors then declare that Chang died, was buried, and was resurrected, after which he retired to the Wudang Mountains to develop Taiji. There he instructed several individuals in both Taiji and spiritual alchemy. The story then skips all the intermediate steps and jumps directly to the Chen Family, who propelled the art into modern times.

From the basic Chang origin story, Yao and Jiang move on to discuss five different origin stories for Taiji, and it is interesting to compare their list of five with an identical, though more-recent, list of five origin stories in Li Xianwu's 1933 book, *Taiji Boxing*. (See review in Volume VI of this series.) While the verbiage differs, the order is the same. One conjecture is that this was a list commonly accepted at the time both these books were written, though it also is possible that Li cribbed from Yao and Jiang's earlier book. Perhaps I'll run across similar lists as I continue to go through *Brennan Translations*' copious catalog of translations of early Chinese Taiji and kung fu texts.

However that may turn out, this list of five origin stories discusses Xu Xuanping of the Tang Dynasty teaching something called the Thirty-seven Postures, the Yu family's Innate Nature Boxing, Cheng Lingxi's fourteen-posture Small Highest Heaven Boxing, Yin Liheng's seventeen-posture Acquired Nature Method, and Chang San-feng's Thirteen Postures. Of course, no one now knows just what these prototype internal styles looked like.

Next, the authors offer short chapters on the natural internal skill of Taiji boxing, the secrets of Taiji, the soul of Taiji, an explanation of Taiji long boxing, and how Taiji, Xingyi, and Bagua are intertwined systems. In this last section, he refers to explanations on this topic by his "colleague Sun Lutang," which is certainly a recommendation. (See Volume IV for reviews of Sun's books.)

The following chapter delves into Taiji's "Four Prohibitions" and "Eight Requirements," each of which is treated to a pithy paragraph. The prohibitions should be familiar to all Taiji players:

1) Using effort and holding your breath
2) Sticking out your chest and kicking out your waist
3) Lifting your shoulders and pulling down your neck
4) Stiffening of the movements

The requirements also should be familiar:

1) Sinking your shoulders and dropping your elbows
2) Drawing up your head top and aligning your crotch
3) Closing your mouth and touching your tongue to your upper palate
4) Containing your chest and loosening your waist
5) Having a pure naturalness
6) Inside and outside joining together
7) Passive and active exchanging roles
8) Seeking stillness within movement

The authors then compare Taiji with hard-style boxing arts, obviously coming down on the side of Taiji. A list of Yang Style postures comes next, and after that are "maps" of the eight directions (Cardinal and Ordinal) and the five steps, here called Five Positions. These aren't really maps, but more on the order of simple charts that don't seem to me to be particularly helpful.

The next topic is Taiji diagrams, including the Zhou Lianxi's earlier and more elaborate diagram as well as the more familiar double-fish diagram. Movement charts follow. I assume that this is an attempt to depict the stepping pattern of the Yang form. I've seen similar charts in other martial arts books, some fairly useful and others ranging from the arcane to the pretty pointless. The charts in this book seem to me to be of the latter sort, even though the authors provide an explanation of them.

Finally the authors come to the form instruction section, presenting a long Yang Style. Unlike the movement charts, the form instruction is much better than most similar efforts in other Taiji books. Occupying more than 200 pages, the instructions are relatively detailed and the photos decent, with the authors trading off duties as models. I'm always skeptical that one can properly learn a martial art from a book, but Yao and Jiang give the instruction section their best shot.

Push hands, here called "playing hands" is the subject of the next chapter, which is led off by a number of Taiji Classics by Wang Tsungyueh and others. After that, the two authors square off in photos of Tui Shou and freeform push hands for several pages of instruction.

The book then ends with about twenty-five pages of additional Taiji Classics, some attributed, some not. Each statement from the Classics is accompanied by an explanatory text that often adds depth to the original work. A critical element in this presentation of the Classics is one that I have only rarely seen but that is interesting and important. It's called "The Twenty-Word Formula," and these twenty words describe different specific types of application: scattering, flashing, carrying, rubbing, reserving, sticking, following, arresting, grabbing, reversing, softening, warding, dragging, breaking, covering, pinching, falling, continuing, pressing, and spreading. Some of these can be linked to the Thirteen Postures, while others are not generally discussed in Taiji books.

All-in-all, *Taiji Boxing Explained* is a very worthwhile read for the Taiji enthusiast, and I highly recommend it for those at the beginner and intermediate stages. More advanced students will appreciate the authors' take on the Taiji Classics.

Essential Concepts of Tai Chi
It is - It is Not - IT IS

by William Ting
(Xlibris/William Ting, 2015, 138 pages)

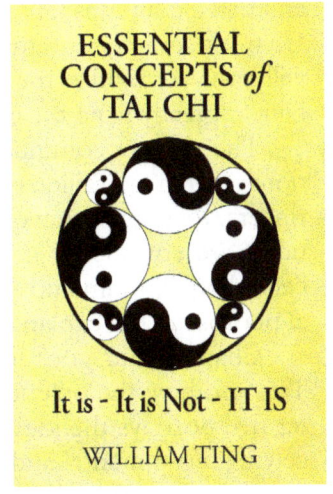

Normally when purchasing an unknown book, one should follow the old adage: "Buyer beware." In the case of William Ting's *Essential Concepts of Tai Chi*, the phrase should be: Buyer be *aware*. Be aware while you're reading, because this book is stuffed with excellent material.

Essential Concepts of Tai Chi opens with eight pages of accolades for Ting's first book, *Answers to Common Tai Chi and Qigong Questions*. I haven't had a chance to read that book, but apparently is consists of sixty-five general questions and answers about Taiji and chi kung. These forewords are followed by a twelve page introduction by one of Ting's students. This has some substance, but like the preceding pages, it is mostly praise for Ting. After a while, all this seems a bit much, but these sections are easily skipped in favor of Ting's own words and ideas.

And excellent words and ideas they are. Chapter one states Ting's purpose for the book and includes why and how he came to learn Taiji. And why he teaches. By the end of this short chapter, I had a good sense of how generous and sincere a teacher he might be, and even this early in the book, it's obvious that he is out to tell you something worth hearing.

Chapter two discusses chi and its relation to life as well as to Taiji. This discussion goes into greater depth on the subject than is the norm among Taiji books, and Ting's inventive metaphors and examples help clarify what is often a difficult subject, particularly for beginning students. Elements touched on are the difference between the "chi" in "Taiji" and "chi" energy, different qualities that chi energy can take (both positive and negative), silk reeling, and awareness, health, and emotions as they affect and are affected by chi.

The next chapter details fundamentals of Taiji practice as they relate to balance, mind, and body. These three aspects are followed by what Ting calls Taiji's "24 Musts," which are important points to adhere to in order to establish correct physical structures and alignments within the Taiji form. In essence, these points are simply concepts from the Taiji Classics that have been recast in plain language and enumerated in ways that highlight their meaning and significance. Each aspect is given ample play, and while experienced Taiji players will easily recognize the importance of these points, beginners can benefit greatly from the clearness of Ting's presentation.

The chapter continues with an explanation of five vital connections within a Taijiquanist's body: shoulders/hips, elbows/knees, fingers/toes, nose/navel, and tailbone/feet. Taiji's three structural bows are considered next, followed by Ting's views on unity and central equilibrium and how these aspects are affected by chi. Several photos aid the explanations.

Chapter four goes into some detail on the use of the mind in Taiji and how the practice of Taiji affects the mind in return. Chapter five portrays the idea of mutual and simultaneous giving and receiving, both mental and physical. Several diagrams show how these ideas can be refined and refined again to create a oneness of action and reaction: a true and subtle interaction.

The dichotomy of flowing and firmness occupies the next chapter. The concept of sung is important here in developing an elastic mental and physical nature in which flow and firmness each have their play, leading to mastery of jin. Emptiness and fullness receive a similar treatment in the following chapter. I especially like the way Ting expands the concept of emptiness/fullness into a living and dynamic three-dimensional structure, where, too often, other Taiji writers talk just about stance and the fault of double-weighting.

Relaxing and expanding in relation to sung is the subject of chapter eight. Ting relates sung not only to sinking, relaxation, and balance, but to feelings of extension and expansion. In this aspect, I was reminded of a similar concept in Robert Chuckrow's *Tai Chi Dynamics* (reviewed above), in which Chuckrow discusses the concept of muscular extension as a more profound practice than simple stretching. To this, Ting adds the idea of feeling as if the body is expanding in all directions—not just along the length of the limbs, but as if the body is constantly radiating outward. It is. This material is excellent and would benefit anyone working to improved their quality of sung.

Chapter nine is titled, "Sink–Turn–Expand." These three elements are not, Ting insists, performed as separate entities but are embodied synergically in any given Taiji movement. If they are not, the form will be disordered and the flow of body and energy will be disrupted, making one's Taiji less effective for health and self-development as well as for self-defense. Ting writes:

> When performed as one, the action of "Sink, Turn, Expand" creates the essence of Sung and Jing.

"It is….It is Not….It is…." is the title of the next chapter, and in it, Ting engages in a somewhat philosophical discussion about how things first appear to be what they are, only later to seem as if they are something more, and finally to reappear as an expanded version of what they alway were. Bruce Lee once said something like:

> Before I studied the martial arts, a punch was just a punch. When my studies began, I realized a punch wasn't just a punch. Now that I have mastered the martial arts, I realize, a punch is just a punch.

The difference is that the punch of experience embodies a great deal more understanding of force, dynamics, angle, etc. than did the punch of inexperience, but it's still a punch.

The real thrust of this chapter is to point out that Taiji is so much more than meets the eye, but that much of modern Taiji does not go beyond the external stage and does not embody the genuine internal substance or power that the art is capable of developing. As he attempts to impart some of that substance, Ting discusses the need for accuracy of form, adequate information about the purpose of the movements, and the way that separation and connection work together. Two related concepts that he goes over are "straight within bend, and bend within straight," and "stillness within motion, motion within stillness." Above all, he says, should be awareness—awareness of oneself, others, and one's situation.

Push hands occupies the next chapter. Ting doesn't go in for explanations and photos of people pushing hands, instead discussing the many benefits of correct push hands practice. The text is philosophical in tone and includes a list of important points separated out for emphasis.

The last chapter talks about "walking Taiji": the practice of walking in Bagua-like circle while performing Taiji movements. Originally developed by Chen Ji-Sheng (1905–1988), walking Taiji, Ting says, can be adapted to any Taiji style. Rather than delineating a specific form in text and photos, the author opts to give pointers for readers to apply the concept to their own Taiji forms. The practice of walking Taiji, he says, is very strenuous, but the rewards of stability, flow, strength, and elasticity are well worth the effort.

The book ends here, and if I have a quibble with it, it's maybe a minor one. I would doubt that Ting would perform a set of Taiji but fail to complete the closing movement. "Close" in Taiji is the movement that brings all your swirling energy back to center and helps sink and coalesce it within the tantien. In an important way, it consolidates all that has come before. But *Essential Concepts of Tai Chi* just ends after the final chapter, leaving me with the feeling that it needed to return to center before I closed the back cover. But maybe that's just because I didn't want the book to end.

A number of reviewers of Ting's first book note the high quality of his prose, and the language in this book is no different. Ting is an excellent writer with a conversational style that makes the book a pleasure to read as well as facilitates the delivery of the information he's trying to impart. As mentioned above, the text is filled with inventive ways to explain the concepts he's trying to get across, all of which aid in understanding even the most abstruse concepts.

All-in-all, Ting has produced a gem of a work that imparts valuable information and ideas in clear prose. *Essential Concepts of Tai Chi* is the kind of book that invites re-reading as well as serving as an excellent reference for the subject. It hovers in the space between philosophy and nuts-'n-bolts books, and to my mind, it is definitely one of the better explanations of the art on the market. It probably is of more use to the intermediate and beginner student than to more experienced practitioners.

My Experience of Practicing Taiji Boxing

"My Experience of Practicing Taiji Boxing"
   (Written in 1929, published in *Wu Zhinqing's Authentic Taiji*, 1936. Brennan Translations, July 2016. 30 pages.)

"On Studying Taiji's Pushing Hands"
   (Written in 1955, two years before Xiang's death and later published within the 1980s reprints of his novels. Brennan Translations, July 2016. 14 pages.)

By Xiang Kairan

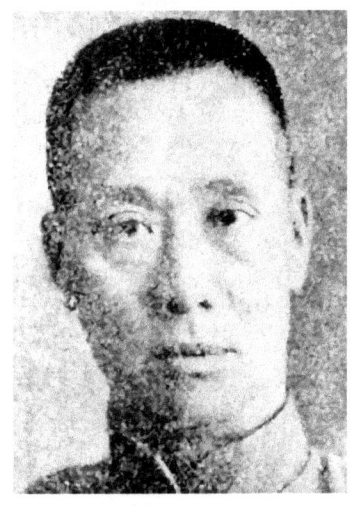

This short book, whose collective title is *My Experience of Practicing Taiji Boxing*, is really two long essays combined into one volume. As the publishing information on them above makes clear, the two were written decades apart. The first, dated 1929, was written when Xiang had practiced Taiji for only four years, which means the latter essay is his take on the art after thirty years of practice. This makes for an interesting bookends look at a practitioner in both the early and late stages of his practice life.

Translator Paul Brennan mentions in passing that Xiang was a novelist. More specifically, Xiang was a writer of Wuxia, the popular Chinese fantasy action-adventure literature containing martial arts stories. Wuxia novels are the genre that spawned kung fu movies and TV shows and are, in many respects, the Chinese equivalent to the American Western. Wuxia stories go back to the roots of kung fu, but in terms of the modern Wuxia novel, Xiang is historically significant.

> Xiang Kairan (pen name Pingjiang Buxiaosheng) became the first notable Wuxia writer, with his debut novel, being *The Peculiar Knights-Errant of the Jianghu*. It was serialized, 1921–1928 and was adapted into the first wuxia film, *The Burning of the Red Lotus Temple* (1928)[1]

The first episode of this movie was directed by Zheng Zhengqiu, and the rest were completed by Zhang Shichuan, both founding fathers of Chinese cinema. It was released from 1928 to 1931 in nineteen feature-length episodes, and runs an astounding total of twenty-seven hours. I'd love to see it, and so would you, but don't bother trying to find a copy. As far as anyone knows, none survive.[2]

The two essays in this book are extremely interesting, but for somewhat different, though linked, reasons. Neither are instructional in nature, but are expository and discuss a number of historical tidbits, principles, and theoretical aspects of Taiji. The relatively early date of the first essay lends modern readers a number of revealing insights into Taiji as it was practiced in the first quarter of the 20th century.

Xiang had earlier studied external kung fu, but his story begins by detailing how he first learned about internal styles of boxing—Bagua, Xingyi, Taiji, and a more obscure style known as Yue School Continuous Boxing—in 1907, oddly while visiting a friend from Hebei who was living at the time in Japan. (See Volume III of this series for a review of a manual by Wang Xinwu on Yue School Continuous Boxing in Volume III of this series.)

He subsequently began searching for teachers of those arts, but it wasn't until 1913 that he met two practitioners of Bagua and Xingyi. In addition to demonstrating their arts for him, these practitioners told him about Taiji, further piquing his interest. He had to wait until 1925, however, while living in Shanghai, when he was fortunate enough to meet and study under Chen Weiming, a leading student not only of Yang Chengfu, but also of Sun Lutang. During the same time,

Xiang also studied under Wang Zhiqun, who had been a student of Wu Chienchuan, son of the founder of Wu Family Taiji.

Working under superb exponents of such disparate backgrounds—Yang, Wu, and Sun—and seeing Taiji performed so differently among them, Xiang became puzzled by the same issues that generations of beginners have pondered ever since: What exactly is Taiji, which forms are "real," and who is doing Taiji correctly?

At this early stage, Xiang figured he was too much the novice to adequately judge any of these practitioners, and before long, he had to leave Shanghai for Hunan. There, he could not find another Taiji teacher, so he contented himself with practicing on his own. In 1928, he followed the Chinese army to Beijing, and though some of the more famous Taiji exponents who had lived there, such as Yang Chengfu and Wu Chienchuan, had already relocated to Nanjing or Shanghai, Xiang did find seasoned practitioners in Xu Yusheng and Liu Enshou whose forms were similar to that taught by Wu Chienchuan, though both men also had studied under Yang Chengfu and Chen Style practitioner Chen Jifu.

Xu recommended that Xiang meet Chen, but according to Xiang:

> It might have been better if I hadn't. After meeting him, I was even more confused than before, because this authentic version of Taiji Boxing is not only entirely different in appearance from Wu Jianquan's teachings, but also completely dissimilar to Yang Chengfu's.

I think it's safe to say that his words echo the confusion most Taiji practitioners experience early on in their Taiji careers. To compound Xiang's puzzlement, all his teachers pushed hands using different patterns and with different emphases. His conclusion at the time was that the Yang version of four-corners was the most complete, with the others missing elements and therefore lacking comprehensiveness.

Xiang's opinion here may be inaccurate, colored by his lack of observing experts other than the few he had already encountered in his four years of practice. Be that as it may, Xiang had, by then, become a firm adherent of Taiji.

> As a result of my personal research into Taiji Boxing, I am deeply convinced as to the meticulousness of the boxing

> theory and the thoroughness of the boxing techniques, and that the practicing of it is a case of pros without cons. Something other boxing arts are not capable of.

I have to insert a similar caveat. While I, too, am convinced of the efficacy, on many levels, of Taiji, I also recognize that many masters of other martial arts also are superlative. A Taiji exponent is only as efficient and adept as his or her experience with the art is long and deep. Real masters are few and far between, and I've seen videos of Taiji "masters" being knocked out in seconds by much younger opponents trained in external fighting arts or MMA. In the end, it's not the art that makes the master. It is the hard work, diligence, and sincere and extensive effort put in over time by a talented individual. And as has often been noted, hard stylists tend to become softer in their approach as they age, and soft stylists become harder in the expression of their energies. Long experience, it seems, leads martial artist from many backgrounds to a comfortable middle ground.

Even Xiang is aware of the shortcomings of Taiji as a martial art.

> After the first martial arts competition in Nanjing [October, 1928], it was noticed that those who specialized in Taiji Boxing often did not win.

He then goes on to try to explain this situation. First, of all the boxing arts, Taiji is the most difficult to apply. This, he says, is due to the lengthy training period required to achieve a high level of proficiency in Taiji as opposed to the external martial arts, many of which can be effectively learned in a fairly short time. This is not because of the relative difficulty of Taiji movements, per se, many of which can be found in other martial styles.

The real reason is that a large part of Taiji's training is teaching one to tap into continuous, circular movement that is developed in and issued from a specific location—the legs—guided in specific ways from another specific location—the waist, which includes the lumbar region—and manifested in various ways in various places in the body, most usually the limb and hands but, just as importantly, from the shoulders, back, and just about everywhere else in the body. Many years—even decades—of practice are required just to begin to recognize these fundamentals in one's own body, stance, posture, and energy flow, and if they are not adhered to in practice until they become fully integrated into the body and its method of movement, then potentially fatal faults will manifest during combat.

Another reason for Taiji's apparent weakness against hard-style opponents, Xiang says, is that most practitioners of other martial arts engage in sparring and actual combat with others, while Taiji's reliance on push-hands as its sole method of combat training can leave a Taiji practitioner—even one who is advanced—at a disadvantage when facing an opponent who has fought often.

To this, I would add another important aspect that Xiang only touches on. Taiji is primarily a defensive rather than an attacking art. It relies on initial input from the opponent, which the Taiji exponent then takes advantage of. But in a ring or combat arena, both fighters must initiate attacks, not just respond to them. Expert Taiji exponents might be able to feint or otherwise cause an opponent to launch an attack to which they can respond, but most Taiji players—even those who are very good—do not have that level of combat sophistication.

Xiang then goes on with a discussion of "double pressure," more commonly known as "double-weighting." He begins this with a quote on the subject from Wang Tsungyueh's *Taiji Boxing Classic*, which concludes that this fault is largely responsible for any failure in the Taiji exponent to successfully neutralize and emit power. Xiang follows this quote with his own take on double pressure, which moves the concept beyond what he considers to be misconceptions of it envisioned by many Taiji practitioners, who limit the idea to avoiding putting equal pressure on both feet. He concludes:

> Even down to a single finger, you still have to distinguish clearly between emptiness and fullness.

Internal power is the subject of the next section, with Xiang discussing the idea that power developed through circular movement is far different from the sort developed by using muscular force, punching bags, and lifting weights. Instead of relying on one or another part of the body to deliver energy, it relies on whole-body power which produces a shocking, rather than slamming, blow.

All of the above principles, he says, are developed by practicing slowly, which allows the individual to carefully observe the body and correct its postures and movements according to Taiji fundamentals.

The author then presents a mini-bio of Chang Sanfeng, which states that Chang was a scholar, a poet, and expert calligrapher and painter. Xiang also states that Chang moved to the mountains after being inspired by the paintings of Ge Zhichuan. These descriptive terms and ideas might well describe Chang, though they are more specific than any I've read before. Most scholars state that little is known of Chang, or even if he actually existed. Xiang's descriptions also clash with the more usual depiction of Chang as sloppy and dirty. Most Taiji people know the legend of Chang, which says he learned Taiji in a dream after watching a fight between a snake and a stork, in which the snake was victorious due to its undulating, evasive movements that kept it from being stuck, then striking back at opportune moments. Xiang foregoes the fight between the snake and stork, but declares that the entity who came to Chang in his dream was the "Dark Warrior Emperor," who translator Brennan clarifies as being a Taoist "god of war."

Following this is a discussion of the three "elixir fields," or tantien, of the human body: the crown of the head, the solar plexus, and the more commonly known area just below and behind the navel. He also goes into the need for the Taijiquanist to utilize abdominal breathing to stimulate this lower tantien. This sort of breathing is not possible, he says, without proper posture and relaxation. Sung!

The next section is a discussion of technique. Xiang is not a fan of Taiji exponents explaining Taiji's functionality through the practice of techniques. In fact, he seems to dislike even considering techniques as viable, and he decries teachers who try to impart elements of Taiji functionality through demonstrations of them. True, Taiji is more of a spontaneous, interpretive art than one that tends to impart specific responses to specifics attacks, but I think that Xiang takes his criticism a little too far here. Even though the techniques he mentions are legitimate within the form, his main observation is, "Good grief!"

Techniques are not the goal of Taiji, but they do exist within the form, and it can be helpful for beginners to see and understand them to get an idea of how Taiji works and how it feels inside while it's working. No practitioner should learn a technique or two for each movement and let it rest at that, especially as many of Taiji's movements contain a great number of possible techniques. Within the simple Grasping Bird's Tail of the Northern Wu Style that I practice, I've found more than twenty-five possible techniques, though admittedly some are variations on a couple of themes. Knowing them allows me to use them. And if I'd never seen how Wild Horse Tosses Mane can be used as a throw, I'd never have been able to use it on a rude fellow who tried to punch me during push hands because he couldn't get to me any other way. (I stopped him from slamming to the ground, but he got the message.)

Learning techniques can give beginners and intermediate students an idea of how Taiji functions, but it also should be stressed that once a technique is learned, it should be largely forgotten. Afterward, the innate knowledge of a technique allows it to spontaneously manifest during sparring or combat—something that would not be possible if potential purposes of the movements are never understood.

The next subject Xiang tackles is the idea of speed in Taiji, which does not mean fast or slow but is embodied in the phrase from the Taiji Classics: "If my opponent moves, I move before him." Thus, speed can be fast or slow, depending on the situation. The point is to match one's own speed to the speed of the opponent's movements. A large part of this is employing "listening energy," which combines accurate and prompt observation with physical sensitivity, and "sticking energy," which allows one to attach oneself to the opponent to take control of his force and appropriately counter his movements.

Xiang's next target for disparagement is the idea that one can add practices from external boxing styles to the benefit of one's Taiji. This, he rightly states, would actually be counterproductive because these external elements would stiffen the body and make it less sensitive, while the goal of Taiji practice it to become relaxed, flexible, lively, and sensitive. Further, hard-style practices emphasize direct muscular force, while Taiji aims at an elastic energy. And finally, the linearity of hard-style exercises would impede the circularity of Taiji.

Diligent adherence to proper Taiji practices, Xiang goes on to say, produces both the right kind of Taiji power and the famous ability of longterm practitioners to root solidly, both of which depend a great deal on centeredness and stability. These characteristics—or their absence—can be experienced during push-hands practice, which is why the practice is so valuable. Push hands not only gives the practitioner the experience of finding errors in one's partner and learning to take advantage of them, but more importantly, it presents the opportunity to analyze and correct errors in oneself, improving the quality of one's overall personal practice.

Xiang points out that many hard stylists will turn their bodies sideways during sparring or a fight. They do this to minimize the area they present to the opponent and to extend their reach with the forward hand. But this is not the Taiji way. Instead, Taijiquanists should directly face the opponent. This allows them to center their bodies and tuck their tailbones, giving their waists free play—a factor essential in eliminating double pressure (double weighting), neutralizing the opponents energy, and delivering full-body power.

Then, in a lengthy and curious passage, Xiang attacks the idea of describing Taiji in terms of "Thirteen Postures." As any serious practitioner knows, the Thirteen Postures are the foundational movements of Taiji, but Xiang criticizes those who describe the postures as foundational. "This is an interpretation," he states, "so forced as to be beyond belief."

Asserting that the Thirteen Postures can only be analyzed through experience in pushing hands, he proposes that they be termed the "Thirteen Dynamics." He further says of the eight postures known as the four Cardinal Directions (Ward Off, Push, Press, and Rollback) and four Ordinal Directions (Shoulder Strike, Elbow Strike, Pull, and Split):

> We can only go as far as calling them "eight kinds of hand techniques" and are really not able to consider them to be "eight postures.... As for the five "postures" of stepping forward, back, left, or right, or staying in the center, this is even more nonsensical and silly.

His reason for this statement is that the idea of five major stepping patterns is a no-brainer. Every martial art utilizes footwork that goes in all the directions as well as staying centered.

Certainly this is true of the five stepping patterns, but it doesn't hurt to codify the idea, particularly for beginners. Perhaps the most applicable idea for Taiji exponents is that Central Equilibrium is the primary stance from which the other four extend. And further, the idea of front and back and left and right help remind the Taijiquanist that any movement in any direction requires a reciprocal movement, no matter how minute, in the opposite direction. This is a simple matter of physics: "For every action there is an equal and opposite reaction." As the Taiji Classics put it, "If there is up, there is down; if there is forward, there is backward." This is an important principle to remember.

As for the eight postures that comprise the four Cardinal and four Ordinal Directions, Xiang proposes that they be considered eight kinds of hand techniques. I think that Xiang is onto something, though I would have stated it differently—and have at length in my book, *Circling the Square: Observations on the Dynamics of Tai Chi Chuan*. Most people do think of these eight elements as postures, but there has to be more to them than that. If they are simply the postures of Taiji, then what about all the movements that aren't one of those eight postures? Needle Sinks to the Bottom of the Sea isn't obviously one of them, nor is Parry and Punch or many others.

So, instead of thinking of these eight forms as postures or even, as Xiang suggests, eight kinds of hand techniques, I believe that we should look at them as something else entirely—especially the four Cardinal Directions, which seem to me to be the true foundation of the art's movements. Every Taiji movement contains at least one of the four Cardinal Directions, which are the four principal ways that the body can act as a unit, and those energies flow through the body to create the many diverse Taiji movements.

Ward Off is the expression of energy, either forward or backward, from one leg into the opposite arm. Push is the expression of energy directly forward or backward, both of which also imply up and down. Press is the expression of energy, either forward or backward, from one leg into the same-side arm. And Roll Back is the expression of energy on a plane around the waist. All of these expressions of energy occur circularly, most commonly in arcs of circles or ovals and often in spirals. Thus, the four Cardinal Directions should really be termed the four Cardinal Energies. The four Ordinal Directions—or Energies—are simply convenient categories into which one can combine one or more of the Cardinal Energies in various ways.

Translator Brennan points out somewhere in the text that Xiang seems to have written this essay without subsequently refining it because it is excessively wordy, somewhat repetitive, and occasionally disjointed. Regarding the latter, the author frequently jumps from one topic to an entirely different one without either logical flow or any sort of segue, and he sometimes takes up the same topic in two separate locations. The next section is a perfect example. Here, Xiang jumps to an anecdote about a Mr. Meng, who excelled at an art called Silken Boxing, which is described as being similar to Taiji in that it was an internal style whose exponents practiced a Taiji-like push hands pattern.

Before he learned Silken Boxing, Meng, who was large and brawny, worked as a bodyguard and was skilled enough with a saber that he gained some fame. He also was an arrogant braggart and know-it-all when it came to the martial arts. One day while staying at an inn, he engaged others in conversation with his usual superior attitude. After a few minutes, an old, white-haired man at another table gave a sneering laugh. Incensed, Meng replied, "Being as decrepit as you are, what would you know about fighting?"

The old man responded:

> Among the mighty are those who are mightier. In martial arts, no one presumes to praise his own abilities. But because you are young, you think you know everything, and so you are unaware of how ridiculous you are.

Completely ticked off, Meng attacked the old man, with the usual consequence in situations like this in tales like this. After the old man thoroughly defeated Meng without doing much of anything at all, Meng begged him to take him on as a student. The old man agreed, and Meng began to learn the thirteen postures of Silken Boxing, but only absorbed eight of them before the old man died. The fact that this boxing had thirteen postures as well as Taiji-like push hands seems to indicate that it was a version of Taiji.

Xiang then goes on to describe two other internal boxing styles —Zimen and Yumen Boxing—both of which also were essentially Taiji. This seems to point to a factor regarding many martial arts, particularly today. That is, many people learn some sort of boxing art, rename it and give it some sort of mystical or pseudo-historical background, and claim they are the sole inheritors and masters of this superlative style. Xiang says they do that to solicit customers, but many also do it to shroud themselves in mystique.

Next, Xiang discusses how difficult it is to learn Taiji, even for those who are dedicated. This difficulty is further exacerbated by other factors. Even qualified teachers often alter or tailor their teachings to particular students. Worse, some of their students learn only partially and then spread a watered-down version of their arts to their own students. These factors lead at best to differences and at worst to deficiencies or distortions and confusion when different students of the same teacher come away with different versions of the teacher's style.

One example Xiang cites is Yang Style:

> Yang Luchan's art is only a hundred years old, but already his teachings are very different from Chen Jifu's. For that matter, Wu Jianquan [Chienchuan] learned from the Yang family, and yet his version is distinct from Yang Chengfu's. Even more peculiar is that Yang Chengfu's elder brother Yang Mengxiang [Shao-hou] learned from the very same family, and yet his Taiji is only practiced as a broken-energy version, each technique expressing power, releasing a vocalized thumping no different from external styles of boxing.... I once asked Chen Jifu if among the practitioners in the Chen Family Village there is a version that practices broken energy. He said there is not.

I've quoted this at length both to show what Xiang meant by forms being altered through time, but also to lead my observations into a discussion of how matters can be misperceived. Certainly Xiang was closer to his sources than I am, but he seems not to fully understand, at this early stage of his own Taiji work, the development of Yang Shaohou's Taiji and, thus, Wu Chienchuan's Taiji. Perhaps he should have asked Chen if Yang Shaohou's energy really was broken since his comments on the subject also highlight what might be misperceptions of those who are not fully aware of how Taiji functions. Remember, Xiang had been practicing for only four years at this time.

To look more deeply into this matter, we have to look more closely at the style practiced by Yang Shaohou. By all accounts, Yang Shaohou, who was Yang Luchan's grandson, did not practice the broad-framed style of Taiji that was passed to and further developed by Yang Chengfu, but instead utilized a small-frame version learned from his father, Yang Jianhou and his uncle, Yang Pan-hou, who was a Manchurian palace guard. It is said that Panhou and Shouhou both preferred the small-frame form because the palace guards wore long, tight-fitting robes, and the small-frame form, with its higher stance, was more suitable for combat in such attire.

This compact version of Yang Style was not well known, and I'm not certain that it's still practiced, at least in that version. Instead, it morphed into Wu Family Style. When Wu Quanyu, founder of Wu Family Style, approached the Yang family for instruction in Taiji, he was not taught by Yang Luchan, it not being proper for a beginning student to learn directly from the current master, at least in the early stages. Instead, Wu was referred to Yang Panhou, who taught him and, eventually, his son, Wu Chienchuan, both of who also were Manchu palace guards. This, then, is the origin of the Wu Family's small-frame style, though the Wu Family has consistently tightened the frame of their style over the years, now making many of its movements almost miniscule. If Xiang believed that Yang Shaohou's form used broken energy, did he also believe that of the style practiced by the Wu family, who learned in part from Shaohou?

There might actually be another explanation for Xiang's belief that Yang Shaohou's style utilized a "broken energy." The smaller the frame, the tighter the circular movements and the more potentially shocking they are. In a truly expert practitioner, those circles can occur entirely within the body and cannot be seen externally. This relative invisibility of Yang Shaohou's circles might account for the belief of some, including Xiang, that his energy was broken. They simply couldn't perceive its internal connectivity.

As for Yang Shaohou's vocalizations and his style seeming to be no different from external styles, consider not only the ability of a higher stance to deliver greater shocking power, but also this from the *Wikipedia* article on him:

> Yang Shaohou was also known to have had a very forceful nature, and both of these masters [the other being Yang

Panhou] are considered to have been very demanding teachers; only interested in teaching those that could stand their tough training regimes....This [small-frame style] was characterized by high and low postures with small movements done in a sometimes slow and sometimes sudden manner. His fajin was hard and crisp, accompanied by sudden sounds. Master Yang Jun described him thus: "The spirit from his eyes would shoot out in all directions, flashing like lightning. Combined with a sneer, a sinister laugh, and the sounds of 'Heng!' and 'Ha!', his imposing manner was quite threatening." During practice with his students, Yang Shaohou was not known for pulling his punches.[3]

So, I have to take with a grain of salt Xiang's criticism that Yang Shaohou exhibited broken energy and was essentially practicing like an external stylist. Taiji develops hardness equally with softness, and by all accounts, Yang Shaohou was a superlative, if vicious, Taijiquanist. But as I've said, despite Xiang's closeness to the sources of the major family styles, he had only been practicing for four years when he wrote this text and might have been ignorant of some of the points I've made above.

In the next section, Xiang discusses several ideas. The first is the propensity for martial artists to usually but wrongfully attribute their art to a mystical past or to a mystical hero. This, he says disparagingly, is part of Chinese culture, which venerates forefathers more than it does people in the present, no matter how talented. But then, ironically, he uses as an example Chang Sanfeng, to whom he has already attributed characteristics and historical facts that are not generally borne out by serious historical research into Chang. And here, he adds additional "facts," namely that Chang passed his art on to Song Yuanqiao, Zhang Songxi, and seven unnamed others. Though he does conclude that there are "no detailed records of his techniques," these are pretty specific details given that Chang might not really have existed, and if he did, there is some confusion about exactly which Chang Sanfeng he might have been among the two or three who are mentioned in the Chinese historical annals of that general time period. Nor is the lineage from Chang to the Chen family at all clear, and the references to potential intermediaries are vague.

Xiang's next point also counters his original statement by reinforcing the idea that one *should* venerate the past when he states that there is a five-word secret in Huang Baijia's *Boxing Methods of the Internal School*. These secrets, Xiang says, are "focused, potent, expedient, sticky, precise," but they are not part of modern Taiji curriculum. These five points are pretty good, but Xiang is essentially giving here a criticism that is similar to the negative criticism of modern films: "They just don't make movies like they used to." Well, no, they don't, at least not technically since film technology has come a long way. But in the past, there were just as many lousy and formulaic movies as there are now, at least percentage-wise—we just ignore and never watch them. And today there are great ones. Likewise, a modern martial arts master is just as much a master as those of the past, overblown myth and legend notwithstanding.

Next, the author launches himself on another round of criticism that seems misplaced. Although previously in the text he often has referred to external and internal boxing, he now scorns the division of kung fu into Shaolin and Wudang. His argument is somewhat convoluted but breaks down like this:

1.) Division and competition produces progress in most human endeavors, but not in the martial arts. His logic for this is that the origins of many Chinese martial arts are obscured by the past and that probably there are many kung fu styles that do not fall into one or the other of these categories, such as those practiced by itinerant martial artists of the past.

2.) Another negative element to division into the two major schools is that practitioners can become segregated by such divisions, with exponents becoming bound by their traditions to the detriment not only of their art, but of kung fu in general. And all too often, he says, this leads to corruption of both tradition and technique by those who have little or partial knowledge. To support this, he cites martial styles that he says are essentially phony and created for the purpose of "advertising," such as Qi Family Boxing and Maitreya Boxing, both of which have questionable pseudo-mystical pasts. "Such people," he says, "have a limited knowledge, as well as a mentality of taking advantage of their forefathers in order to advertise themselves, a flaunting that cannot be admonished enough."

Regarding the first, I take his point, but the point does not logically follow from the criticism. And further, I agree that there are a great many martial arts that combine both soft and hard techniques—most often utilizing soft-style defense with hard-style offense. Perhaps we do need middle ground terminology between Shaolin and Wudang to accommodate these types of martial arts, which also include some that were developed in other Eastern countries, such as Japanese Kenpo and Hapkido, both of which owe a debt to Taiji, and Javanese Silat, which emphasizes defensive flexibility and liveliness. That's not my call to make, but I do think that there is a fundamental difference in how external-style martial arts—even those with soft-style defenses—function as opposed to internal styles. Xingyi is a good example. It is a very hard style, but it also is very internal.

Regarding the second point, it seems to me that humankind has no dearth of people throughout history whose rigid thinking cannot allow them to see the worthiness and excellence in others and who rely solely on their own cult of personality to give them emotional and psychological sustenance. Nor is there an end to scam artists. Just as we have plenty of them today, there were plenty in the ancient past of every country, region, and culture. There's always somebody out to make a quick buck or yen off the weak, the foolish, the naive, the fearful, and the desperate. Those seeking martial arts knowledge, whatever the style, tradition, or level of advancement, will come across many such in their quest. So be it. That is the flawed nature of humans and of the world in an imperfect reality. Caveat emptor.

Xiang then launches into a discussion of neutralizing and issuing power by quoting a criticism that he heard said by people who might be even less knowledgeable in Taiji than he was at this stage.

> Yang Chengfu is good at shooting people away but not good at neutralizing, whereas Wu Jianquan is good at neutralizing people but not good at shooting them away. Therefore both of these men have a shortcoming, but if they

were strong in both qualities, then they would be at the peak of Taiji skill.

Responding to this criticism, Xiang writes:

> It happens that some people possess the theory but really cannot understand its reasoning. Issuing and neutralizing only seem to be two things but are actually one, so you cannot issue without being able to neutralize, nor neutralize without being able to issue.

Above I criticized Xiang for seeming to be unaware that Yang Shaohou's circles were most likely so internalized that a viewer only observing his external movement might mistake his energy as being "broken," but here, Xiang does not commit a similar error and is spot on. He explains that different experts are, first and foremost, different people with different builds, temperaments, and proclivities. Yang Chengfu, being a big, beefy guy, was fond of exhibiting his issuing power by shooting people away, while Wu Chienchuan had a polite temperament that was gentlemanly and urbane, and he was not inclined to antagonize his opponents and so usually just neutralized their attacks without bothering to shoot them away.

Xiang concludes that, although he attempted to meet both men when he moved to northern China, by then, both had moved south. Thus he had no opportunity to personally witness or feel their skills.

In the final section of this portion of the book, Xiang moves on to discuss several Taiji principles, such as continuous flow, sinking the energy, and paying attention to the active and passive. He then has some words concerning differences in form between styles and says that these differences are merely superficial as long as the forms adhere to principles of Taiji.

Next in the volume is the second essay, "On Studying Taiji's Pushing Hands," which Xiang wrote in 1955 after studying Taiji for about thirty years. While the previous long-form essay contained some naiveté, it also presented some interesting historical aspects and showed some remarkable insights into basics principles of the art. This later essay delves, as the title states, into pushing hands, and it, too, is insightful—and a little little less naive and more cohesively written.

Interestingly enough, the author starts off by praising something he disparaged in the first essay: the Thirteen Dynamics. Or rather, let me rephrase that. In the previous essay, he disparaged the Thirteen Postures, which he believed were false and limiting categories. But in recasting them as the Thirteen Dynamics, he can praise them as foundational to Taiji and to pushing hands. I went into detail on that above, and while I still think Xiang does not go far enough in his recasting, at least he's on a better track than simply thinking of the "Thirteen" as "Postures." Taiji's solo set is foundational to push hands, he says, but the Thirteen Dynamics are foundational to both.

To further explain Taiji principles, Xiang turns to that tried-and-true wellspring: the Taiji Classics. For the next six pages, he presents important principles from the Classics then explicates each with a paragraph or two of commentary. I won't go into his commentaries, but here are the major categories he explores:

1) The soft and smooth versus the hard and coarse
2) Matching speed of response to the opponent's speed of attack
3) Keeping one step ahead of the opponent in both defense and attack
4) Sensitivity
5) Understanding, or, knowing the opponent while not letting him know you
6) Single-weighting vs double-weighting
7) Sticking and yielding
8) The exchange of passive and active
9) Spontaneous response versus planned response
10) How to issue power
11) The Thirteen Dynamics

The author then goes into the rationale behind pushing hands, followed by descriptions of four principal types and discussions of each:

1) Single-hand fixed-step
2) Double-hand fixed-step
3) Moving-step
4) Large rollback

Each, he says, must adhere to the principles of Taiji, no matter what school-generated variations might exist in the patterns. "Practice a lot over a long time," he writes, "and you will have a breakthrough."

Next he relates his own personal journey in learning push hands. His first teacher, Chen Weiming, was fond, like his teacher, Yang Chengfu, of crowding in with Ward Off and Press, though Chen did not issue power but simply caused Xiang to become stuck and unable to yield. Xiang next worked with Wang Zhiqun (here called Wang Runsheng), and when he tried Chen's crowding tactic, Wang simply disrupted the attack, leaving Xiang off balance. Xiang asked Wang what kind of attacking Wu Chienchuan performed, and Wang answered:

> Wu hardly ever attacks. But if you tried some method of attacking him, he would right away cause you to be unable to use any power or hardly even move.

Wang gave Xiang a succinct lesson in opening and closing during both form practice and push hands. Flicking a handheld fan open and closed, he asked Xiang what was causing the opening and closing. "Your hand," Xiang replied, but Wang shook his head and pointed to the fan's hinge. "It requires this thing in order to be able to open and close." Then he pointed to a door and said, "The door also needs a hinge to open and close" The Taiji hinge Wang was referring to is the waist. Further, the commands for the waist come from the lumbar region, which also supplies Taiji's centeredness.

Xiang's next push hands teacher was Xu Yusheng, of the little-known Song school of Taiji. His push hands focused on opening and closing, coordinating the breath with each movement. Because Xu emphasized the Thirteen Dynamics in both the solo practice and push hands, Xiang says, "his pushing hands exhibited the greatest capacity for using the movement from the solo set."

One of Xu's Song Style brothers, a Mr. Liu, was different. Liu's push hands was very light and then suddenly heavy, very close then very far away, rendering Xiang incapable of either connecting and following or sticking and adhering.

Sometimes he would abruptly lift, and I would be lifted up all the way down to my heels. Sometimes he would abruptly withdraw, and I would topple forward into emptiness. (p. 41)

After Xiang grew savvy to Liu's lures, he would sometimes lash out with external-style techniques only to be admonished:

Pushing hands is a kind of training method, not sparring. You can't have a competitive mentality. It's not about win or lose.

And with the following statement, Xiang closes the essay:

There are many practitioners of Taiji Boxing and many books about it, but texts focusing on theory, especially pushing hands theory, which give a systematic exploration, an endeavor of research recorded for all to study, are still too rare. Thus I have written this piece to supply Taiji Boxing aficionados with some reference material.

Despite its brevity, this has to be one of the best Taiji books that I have yet read from translator Paul Brennan's collection. It transcends the typical Taiji manual to deliver interesting historical insights into the art in China from the early to mid 20th centuries. It also has many excellent and helpful hints on the practice of both the solo form and push hands. Despite my many criticisms of the work, I consider it to be thought-provoking and of great value.

Notes
1 "Wuxia." *Wikipedia*, https://en.wikipedia.org/wiki/Wuxia
2 "The Burning of the Red Lotus Temple." *Wikipedia*, https://en.wikipedia.org/wiki/The_Burning_of_the_Red_Lotus_Temple
3 "Yang Shao-hou." *Wikipedia*, https://en.wikipedia.org/wiki/Yang_Shao-hou

A Study of Taiji Boxing

By Long Zixiang
(Originally published 1952. *Brennan Translations*, 2018, 268 pages)

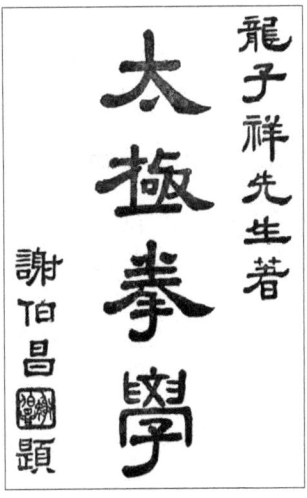

A Study of Taiji Boxing is an involved work with many aspects. I wish I could say it is "by" the purported author, Long Zixiang, but that would be misleading. Long might be responsible for the lengthy form instruction section, but almost all of the rest of the text is lifted verbatim from around a dozen books by other authors, most of which are available from *Brennan Translations*. There are two saving graces to Long's cribbing. First, almost all the sources he's taken material from are excellent and written by high-level practitioners. Second, the material itself is important, and perhaps Long would not have been capable of disseminating it as well as the original authors. The major downside is that, if you've read much Republican Era Chinese martial arts literature, you might have read all this before in its original publications.

I suppose a long book—especially one on any type of kung fu—has to start off with prefaces, and this one is no different. And there are a lot of them. They begin with sixteen poetic inscriptions followed by seven prefaces, only the last of which is by the author. The prefaces by others all are similar: extolling the virtues of the martial arts, especially Taiji, and the skill of the author. There also is a bit of biographical information on the author.

Long began his martial arts career under Tan San (Chow Li Fut) and Gu Ruzhang (Northern Shaolin and Taiji). At the time of the writing of the book, Long was director of the martial arts section of the Hong Kong Chinese Fitness Association and head teacher of the the Kowloon Chamber of Commerce Taiji Boxing Club.

The book begins with a few general remarks. This is the one that resonates the most:

> Taiji theory is mostly the same from master to master, but there are different essentials to be learned from each. The purpose is for you to gain an abundant knowledge of the art. Although the content of such texts can sometimes seem repetitive, you should tirelessly delve into them over and over, and in this way you will be able to examine the views of many masters rather than focus on only one. All those who have contributed to Taiji are to be referenced.

Another remark deals with the inclusion of the other texts:

> Of the extra texts sought our for inclusion in this book, some were left out or merely quoted from, some have been given added commentary for easier interpretation, and some were helpful for making the lineage chart and the [Eight Trigrams] charts. Effort has been made to appropriately fit them within the structure of the book and so those that seem oddly placed are included as "additional texts."

I might complain more about Long's cribbing, but the quality of the information he's copied is too good to pass up.

The main text leads off with the Taiji Classics attributed to Chang Sanfeng. Each is treated to a translation and a commentary. The same goes for the next few Classics—those by Wang Tsungyueh. The next chapter is one of those "added texts," namely the preface from Sun Lutang's *A Study of Taiji Boxing*. (See Volume IV of this series for a review.) This covers primordial energy, the active and passive aspects of reality, and the basic history of Bodhidharma (Damo) bringing the seeds of chi kung and the martial arts to the Shaolin Temple. It also discusses strength versus power and a number of other Taiji precepts, but in general terms.

The next chapter is "Gu Rushing's Experiences of Practicing Taiji Boxing," which is copied from Gu's 1936 manual. After some general remarks, Gu addresses several principles of practice:

1) Loosen
2) Open
3) Extend
4) Tighten
5) Slackness
6) Slow down

Each of these is treated to some depth.

The next chapter is Hu Pu'an's "The Value of Taiji Boxing in Physical Education," which is copied from Wu Zhiqing's 1936 manual. (See review later in this volume.) This piece explains the name of the art, describes its principles of movement, and discusses its value as physical education. The principles are:

1) Your body should be loose.
2) Your energy should be firm.
3) Your spirit should be concentrated.

Another "additional text" comes next, this one a biography of Chang Sanfeng taken from Wu Tunan's 1931 manual, *A More Scientific Martial Art: Taiji Boxing*. (See Volume VII of this series for a review.) This bio contains a lot of specific detail on Chang Sanfeng that probably isn't actually true since most martial arts historians can't determine if Chang actually lived or exactly which Chang Sanfeng he was, since apparently there are several in the historical records, none of which mentions a martial arts connection. I'm inclined to take this account as almost entirely apocryphal.

A far shorter bio of Wang Tsungyueh follows, also copied from Wu Tunan's 1931 manual. Then Huang Chuyin takes up the pen to provide a bio of the book's author, Long.

A Taiji lineage chart is next, although it isn't really a chart but a list. It takes in many of the apocryphal branches of Taiji as it developed through the centuries as well as the more well-known ones, such as the branch that begins with Chang Sanfeng. It also speaks to more modern and historical lineages, such as Li Jingling/Sun Lutang→Gu Ruzhang→author Long Zixiang and others.

More copied text follow, beginning with, "Discussing the Similarities and Differences between Various Versions of the Taiji Boxing Solo Set," copied from Wu Zhiqing's 1936 manual, *Authentic Tai Chi* (reviewed previously in this volume). The explanation here is fairly superficial. Next is "Essentials of Practicing the Taiji Boxing Art," copied from Chen Weiming's 1925 manual. The ten essentials are:

1) Forcelessly press up your head top.
2) Contain your chest and pluck up your back.
3) Your waist must loosen.
4) Distinguish clearly between empty and full.
5) Sink your shoulders and drop your elbows.
6) Use intention, not exertion.
7) Your upper and lower body coordinate with each other.
8) Inside and out join with each other.
9) The movements are linked together without interruption.
10) Within movement, seek stillness.

All of these points are important, and each of them is adequately discussed.

"Taiji Boxing's Five-Word Formula," by Li Yiyu, lists the five and describes each:

1) The mind is calm.
2) The body is lively.
3) The energy is collected.
4) The power is complete.
5) The spirit is gathered.

The Taiji Classic known as the *Song of the Thirteen Postures*, or some such variation on that, is featured next, and after that is "The Trick to Raising and Releasing," by Li Yiyu. This is followed by "Taiji Boxing's Process of Command and Obey," taken verbatim from Wu Tunan's *A More Scientific Martial Art: Taiji Boxing.* (Reviewed in Volume VI of this series.)

1) The lower back is the first to command.
2) The throat is the second to command.
3) The solar plexus is the third to command.
4) The elixir field is the first to obey.
5) The palms are the second to obey.
6) The soles of the feet are the third to obey.

Also from Wu's book comes this list of sixteen important points:

1) Liveliness lies with your waist.
2) Inspiration penetrates to your head top.
3) Spirit courses through your spine.
4) Flowing lies with your energy.
5) Movement lies with your legs.
6) Pressing is felt at the foot.
7) Wielding lies with your palms.
8) Sufficiency reaches to your fingers.
9) Gathering is a matter of your marrow.
10) Arriving is a matter of your spirit.
11) Concentration depends on your ears.
12) Breathing occurs through your nose.
13) Breathing operates from your abdomen.
14) Springiness lies with your knees.
15) Simplify things by using your whole body.
16) Issuing is expressed at every hair.

A discussion of the Eight Gates and Five Steps (the Thirteen Postures/Dynamics) follows but doesn't add much. Then it's on to the form instruction section depicting Yang Style. This occupies about 160 pages, and the textual instructions are fairly good and include function as well as form. The photos, while not great, are adequate and have arrows to indicate the direction of movement. Footwork charts sometimes accompany the photos.

More copied material follows, beginning with "Discussing Playing Hands," by Wu Tunan, and this moves on to "Taiji Boxing's Pushing Hands Curriculum," by Gu Rushing. The former is relatively slight, but the latter has more meat and discusses a number of important aspects, including the three stages of progress in pushing hands. The first stage entails:

1) Open and close, passive and active
2) Sticking, adhering, connecting, and following
3) Hardness and softness, smoothness and coarseness
4) Quickness and leisure, sticking and yielding

The second stage includes

1) Lightness
2) Heaviness
3) Being centered rather than leaning
4) Neither slanting nor digging in
5) Nimbleness

Stage three includes:

1) Weighing energy
2) Neutralizing energy
3) Drawing in

More unattributed Taiji Classics follow, leading into another chapter by Li Yiyu on essentials of practicing the solo set.

The next chapter is an elucidation of the Eight Gates, showing how each can be used in self-defense. The text is okay, but the photos are nearly unidentifiable. The instructions for each posture include the main action, points for attention, and further explanations that suggest other techniques. These end the book.

What a mess this book is, but it's a glorious mess filled with superior information—even if almost all of it comes from other authors. But as I said at the outset, these other authors are experts who have written their own manuals. I can't say that you could read Long's book and get everything of importance from those other authors, but Long sure was selective in what he appropriated. And to give him credit, it's all attributed, so he's not actually guilty of plagiarism, only of calling himself an author rather than an editor.

Taiji Peng
Root Power Rising

by Scott Meredith
(Scott Meredith, 2014, 134 pages)

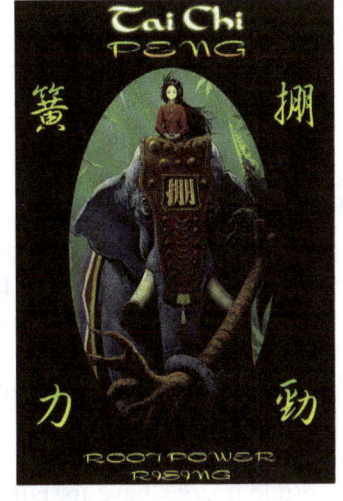

The proliferation of Taiji literature since the 1950s has produced a wide variety of books on various aspects of the art, some overarching, some focused. Most Taiji books are straightforward explications of form, principles, and other aspects of Taiji, while a few are fairly idiosyncratic. That doesn't mean bad, just different in one way or another. Scott Meredith's *Tai Chi Peng: Root Power Rising* is one of those.

Meredith is the author of several books on the martial arts: *JUICE: Radical Taiji Energetics*, *Radical Xingyi Energetics*, and *Tai Chi SURGE*, among them. The reason that some of the words are all-capped in the titles is that they are acronyms for specific principles that Meredith highlights. I haven't yet read his other books, so I'll let those acronyms go for the moment to focus on the one he introduces in this book: RIDE, as in "ride the energy." RIDE stands for Recognize, Initiate, Direct, and Extend. To seasoned Taijiquanists, this is clearly another way of encouraging the exponent to sense incoming force, meet it without resistance, attach to it, alter its path, and move it away (into emptiness, for example).

Meredith states that all the theoretical and conceptual background on chi is contained in his previous *JUICE*, while the purpose of this book is to give the reader tools to sense, open to, empower, and direct chi energy in the body, the result of which is the ability to express Peng energy.

After the introduction, Meredith opens with a chapter titled "Tai Chi and PENG Energy." The description of Taiji is not meant to be all-encompassing but rather a springboard into the concept of Peng. Here, he describes Peng energy mostly through anecdotal evidence of its effects and other aspects rather than more specifically as a compressed and directed wave of chi channeled through specific bodily alignments.

The next chapter discusses Peng energy more deeply, again through anecdotes interspersed with conceptual ideas that don't directly define what the energy is or how it arises. There is some good material here, but the actual definition of Peng remains a little hazy.

With a title like "Energetic Architecture," the next chapter promises a little more directness, but Meredith starts by quoting a Taiji Classic that he states is not generally found in published versions (of which there a great many, at this point). The problem is, he gives no provenance for the quote—either specific source or author—except to say that "it's all over the Chinese internet." "All over the Chinese internet" isn't much of a footnote in terms of information retrieval. Or genuineness, since there's all sorts of BS all over the Internet. Really, if you're going to cite a source as a little known Taiji Classic, that source ought to be both substantial and accessible. Provide a footnote so that I, too, can find this little-known Classic.

Mostly, this chapter is an exegesis of the unsourced Taiji Classic. While it does have its fair share of good information, that good information is buried in an equal amount of hazier material. As I read along, I had the feeling of wandering through a fog, coming upon an object that I could closely examine with interest, then wandering off through the fog again, seeking another object.

The fog here isn't indeterminate information but a degree of obviousness mixed with repetition and slightly off-kilter writing. For example:

> I talked about dropping energy from the dantian to the feet. Subsequently, the dantian refills from below. That's an amazing sensation that tells you you're really getting somewhere. You'll feel the energy come from the soles of the feet, up through your legs, and then it surges up into, not only the

> dantian, but the entire area of the lower hips and abdomen. That's the beginning of the upward process. So the dantian is again important, when the energy comes back around.

Let's rewrite the last part of that passage to eliminate the grammatical and sequential errors:

> You'll feel the energy drop from the dantian, located in the lower abdomen, then rebound up through your legs. From there, it surges into the hips and back into the dantian. That's the beginning of the upward process. [Actually, aren't we now at the half-way mark?] So the dantian is again important when the energy comes back around.

Meredith doesn't really say why this is important, although is it important in the same way that it was important before, which Meredith says is because the dantian is "where energy accumulates from all sources" And further, I think that this concept of the tantien as an accumulator of chi is erroneous. Instead, I believe—with some scientific backing—that the tantien is the generator of chi. The sensation of "storage" comes from development of the tantien to such a degree that the chi it generates is highly refined, powerful, well-directed through open channels (meridians), and instantaneously available. (See my book *The Wellspring: An Inquiry into the Nature of Chi* for a more thorough discussion of this matter.)

The next chapter covers energy hotspots, which are significant acupuncture points through which chi flows or where it has major branches. The information here is good, and Meredith carries the energy all the way through the circuits of the Microcosmic Orbit and the Macrocosmic Orbit to the fingertips, which he says "will feel like bubble wrap when you do this stuff right." By this I take it to mean that the fingers will feel somewhat puffy or pneumatic, not like they're covered in huge blisters.

Next, Meredith takes us through a number of exercises and postures that encourage relaxation and chi flow. In the introductory material to these sections, he states:

These postures have only ever been perfectly demonstrated by one man, the founding creator of this system, Professor Zeng Manqing [Cheng Man-ching].

Really? Out of all of Taiji history, only Cheng could stand perfectly in Ward Off or Golden Rooster on Single Leg? And while Cheng did formulate a thirty-seven movement version of Taiji—which Meredith calls ZMQ37—the postures in that sequence are from Yang Style, though sometimes with variations. Cheng certainly was important to Taiji history and achievement, particularly in the United States, and ZMQ37 deserves recognition as its own distinct style rooted in Yang Style—as is Wu Family Style. But masterful as he was, Cheng was neither the most important nor, probably, the most skillful and powerful fighter in Taiji history. In other words, lots of masters can "perfectly demonstrate" numerous Taiji and chi kung postures. That's why they're masters.

The first drill Meredith shows consists of waving a straight sword back and forth in front of the body at waist height. There are details on how this is done correctly and for what purpose. The next seven postures come straight from Yang Style (ZMQ37): Golden Rooster on Single Leg, Separate Leg, Repulse Monkey, Raise Arms, Wardoff, Single Whip, and Weaving Lady. The idea is to hold these poses with sung (sinking) and correct, non-stressful alignments, so that the body can relax into them and allow one to sense the chi flowing through the body.

The following chapter discusses the idea of single- and double-weightedness, including the differences in adjusting the percentages of how the weight falls: 100/0, 80/20, and 70/30. The chapter after covers what Meredith calls the Relaxation Protocol. Simply, this is holding the poses previously mentioned while a partner supports the weight of any raised limb, such as the leg in Separate Leg or the upraised arm in Golden Rooster. At first, the partner supports most of the weight of the limb but gradually lets off as the poser internally adjusts his or her weight and balance to accommodate for the slackening support.

Finally, two-thirds of the way through the book, the author gets down to the nuts-'n-bolts of Peng. The material in this chapter is easily the best in the book, though some of the preceding material was necessary predicate for what's found here. Before this, he's really just talked about learning to sung and feel the flow of chi. Now he likens Peng to two sorts of surges of energy: the soft wave and the hard wave. Seasoned practitioners will know these well, but Meredith is obviously speaking to those who do not yet, or just barely, feel it. He discusses these two ways to express energy in some detail, stating rightly, for example, that it is generally possible to understand and generate the hard wave more readily that it is to correctly generate the soft version.

An interesting series of drawings illustrates the way one can send a wave of energy rippling up from the feet, through the legs and body, to the hand. I like to observe—and appreciate—the various ways photographers and illustrators try to instill a sense of movement to still images, and this is, for me, a new take that has merit. In these drawings, the final posture is Single Whip, and the energy is shown being generated in the left foot, rippling part way up the left leg before also rippling just a moment later up the right leg. From there, the ripple engages the waist and hips and then the torso before terminating in the arms. I don't know about you, but for me, the initial impulse for Single Whip comes from the right leg, not the left. While the left also reacts to the impulse, it's a sinking that occurs almost simultaneously with the pulse has been generated by the right foot and passed through the waist. But maybe that's just me.

Next Meredith talks about zhanghuang, or the practice of holding energizing postures for long periods of time. This is, essentially, still chi kung. In this case, the postures are the seven poses detailed earlier. Meredith suggests repeatedly "deflating" the postures about 20 percent by controlled slumping, then gradually "inflating" them until they are at full height to help the practitioner make micro-adjustments to stance, alignment, and so forth to encourage a more powerful manifestation of the posture. This would be something akin to performing the Relaxation Protocol on one's own body, and it sounds useful.

Cloud Hands occupies the next chapter, which takes the ideas garnered from the static postures above and sets them into motion. Cloud Hands, Meredith asserts, is one of the most important Taiji movements, and in this, I couldn't agree more. The reader also might check out *The Internal Structure of Cloud Hands* by Robert Tangora (reviewed next), which delves deeply into the refinement of Central Equilibrium through the practice of Cloud Hands. Meredith describes in some detail the movement of the ZMQ37-version of Cloud Hands and how the energy flows through it. I don't do this version of Taiji, or even another version of Yang Style, but no matter. The principles, basic movements, and sensations hold true in my form, too.

In the next chapter, the author forays into personal territory, beginning with the question of what is the difference, if any, between Taiji and chi kung. From there he goes into the various reasons a person might choose to dedicate the time and effort required to really "practice" Taiji and gain the many benefits that accrue from expending that time and effort. For him, in the end, Taiji is art for art's sake. That doesn't mean he eschews the martial, exercise, health, and other benefits that Taiji imparts. Clearly he doesn't. It's just that all of these aspects, because they are so disparate, can find culmination only in the constant if ultimately futile striving for perfection and in blending the movements and the energetics into something that is at once useful, beautiful, and meaningful.

A pretty worthless chapter follows: "The Graphic Taiji Classic." Once you get past the jokey "finding the ancient Taiji essay in a hot pepper shop" shtick, you wind up with five full-page illustrations, each of a Taiji posture and another element, say a panther or a feather, that supposedly is meaningful with regard to the posture. The drawings are by Jeremy Ray, who provides most of the fairly numerous illustrations throughout the book. Ray uses an anime-style of drawing—a style I'm not overly fond of. But at least his figures are well proportioned and executed and are adequate through most of the book. But well executed or not, they don't illuminate anything here that couldn't be shown better by a real human expert doing the modeling. Okay, the drawings aren't completely devoid of meaning, but all they, along with their explanatory text, really do here is occupy nine pages that I think could have been put to better service.

The book ends with a short epilog that might correctly assess the scenario of despair of our times—times in which Taiji might be needed more than ever but in which, Meredith says, post-humans will make the art obsolete.

As I said, this is an idiosyncratic book.

The author writes in a breezy style with occasional exuberant—even hyperbolic—outbursts. For example:

> The full energy cycle…both begins and ends with the energy buzzing and humming in your relaxed dantian; feeling like you have a radioactive beehive down there.

That's pretty floridly descriptive, though it doesn't describe what I feel in my tantian, which is a smoothly rolling ball of energy that is synchronized with my abdominal breathing and sends pulses of energy up my spine and onward into my limbs. I would take any sensation of a radioactive apiary to indicate that the energy is repeatedly hanging up or being constricted while it cycles instead of flowing smoothly. An unconstricted throat does not hum.

I could have been annoyed by Meredith's style, and above I have taken exception with some elements of it. But in the end, I choose to think of it as being his half of a conversation, and I can be prone to exuberant and ungrammatical outburst, myself.

But a more telling criticism is that I don't think that Meredith adequately explicates the subject indicated by the title. The exercises he gives are more about facilitating and directing chi flow, and Peng is so much more than the flow of chi, even if surging chi is what underlies Peng. Equally important are how to amplify the chi flow so that it can produce a wave, how the wave can be directed into different body parts, and how certain areas of the body can be used to control and direct the wave in specific ways, much of which is barely covered here. This is what he should have used those nine pages for, rather than occupying them with cute anime drawings.

In fact, the flowing sensations Meredith often defines as Peng are what I'd call just basic chi flow. If you hold the posture Standing Post, the force you feel coursing through you isn't Peng but chi. It's the same when you hold the postures in Meredith's book. Holding the postures is basic standing chi kung and can encourage chi to flow in certain ways. But chi only becomes Peng when it is given a surging impetus by mind intent and moves into and fills a posture. It seems to me that Meredith constantly conflates the two, but in truth they are not the same. Peng is a dynamic manifestation—a manipulation of chi. Applying that dynamic manifestation in particular ways is to fa jin—to manifest Taiji's power on a physical level in one of a great variety of ways, some yielding, some forceful.

But rather than saying Meredith covered things wrong, I'd say he just didn't cover them enough. This isn't a bad book, and it would definitely be useful to those readers who are feeling the first twinges of chi and are deliberately making forays into that territory. Perhaps for them, the several exercises might assist in further developing their sensations and control of chi, just as any internal-type of chi kung will. But for more experienced practitioners who can generate and, to some extent or other, control the chi flow and its manifestation as Peng energy, most of the material in these pages will be familiar, and maybe even weak.

But there are a couple of aspect about this book that help redeem it. First is its exuberance. Meredith clearly loves Taiji and is excited to talk about it. That excites me, too. And the exercises and techniques he describes worked for him in discovering his power, so they'd probably work for you, too. Also his assessment of Taiji as a total living art form resonates with my own approach. And finally, despite some occasional hyperbole, he manages to convey the sensation of chi flow and ways to make that flow stronger as well as more tangible.

And like he says, once you feel it, well....

The Internal Structure of Cloud Hands
A Gateway to Advanced T'ai Chi Practice

by Robert Tangora
(Blue Snake Books, 2012, 142 pages)

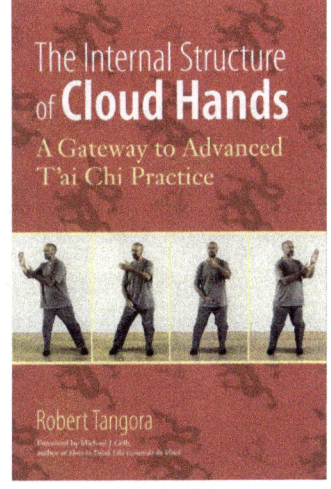

Most nuts-'n-bolts Taiji books try to break down and closely examine the dynamics of body movement, energy flow, and other aspects of Taiji by looking at the broader picture. These are the astronomers, gazing with telescopes into the macro structure of the universe. And then there are the rare ones, like *The Internal Structure of Cloud Hands* by Robert Tangora, that are just the opposite. In these, the authors gaze with microscopes into the finer and more hidden details of the art.

The focus in this book, obviously, is very sharp. In fact, it could be said to be almost infinitely fine because the actual subject is what is commonly called Central Equilibrium, which the author usually refers to by its Chinese term: "zhong ding." He also delves into what he terms cross-body power and left/right alignment or joint power to help explicate zhong ding. He accomplishes this by concentrating on a single movement from the Taiji form. From the introduction:

> Of the thirteen postures in the T'ai Chi Classics, Cloud Hands is the stepping method of zhong ding. This stepping method is the fundamental stepping method in t'ai chi ch'uan because it embodies the internal process of stepping,

turning, and weight shifting regardless of the direction of the step.... Thus, Cloud Hands is a paradigm for the internal symmetry in t'ai chi ch'uan through the hidden relationship between the stepping method, the changes of nei chin, and cross-body power.

I'll deal with the problem with this statement before moving on to praise. Tangora refers to Cloud Hands as one of the Thirteen Postures of the Taiji Classics, conflating it with Central Equilibrium, but this is manifestly not so. The Thirteen Postures are: Five Steps (Central Equilibrium, Step Left, Step Right, Step Forward, Step Backward), four principal energies (Ward Off, Rollback, Press, Push), and four ancillary energies (Shoulder Strike, Elbow Strike, Split, and Pull/Pluck), and I don't see Cloud Hands among them. Although there are a few nearly pure expressions of Central Equilibrium and the four principal energies within the form, most Taiji movements combine multiples of these thirteen "postures." In my parsing, Cloud Hands employs three: Rollback, Ward Off, and Step Left (or Right if you're doing a lefthand form). Some readers might think I'm nitpicking here, but just as it's important not to slur your movements while performing the Taiji form, it's also important not to slur your ideas when discussing Taiji—or anything else.

Aside from this one gaffe, this book is top-notch. Most of the text throughout is an extended discussion, explanation, and expansion of the concepts referred to in the quote above. Along the way, Tangora presents a number of practical exercises—primarily chi kungs—to empower one's awareness of zhong ding and to energize movements surrounding it. There are plenty of diagrams and photos to illustrate the exercises and other important points. The purpose, Tangora stresses, is to refine one's awareness of zhong ding in such a way that the "radius" of one's central equilibrium shrinks to, ideally, an infinitesimally small axis. The smaller the axis of rotation, the more effective your Taiji will be, regardless of your purpose in practicing.

Related subjects that are covered include a discussion of the proper functioning of the waist and legs, bouncing to initiate the vertical component of cross-body power, and the basic zhong ding stepping method. Next is a chapter on left and right alignments in Cloud Hands, which includes the concept of opening and closing the body or various body parts and how the jin changes during Cloud Hands and with the weight shifts

Harmonizing cross-body power and left/right alignment power is the subject of the next chapter, which focuses on twisting and spiraling, including reeling silk energy. Opening and closing the lower body and stepping are briefly covered next, leading into an informative chapter on Taiji's bow energy.

Rooting is discussed in the next chapter, and following that, is a chapter on rolling the chi energy ball. I've found that this is one of the quickest ways to get beginners to feel chi energy. After that are chapters on zhong ding energy, spinal alignment, and how energy spirals through the Cloud Hands movements. A chapter on sung—that special Taiji term that denotes relaxation, sinking, and so much more—includes practical observations on how to initiate internal energy movement with the mind.

This leads naturally into a chapter on the internal separation of yin and yang, and that into a chapter on harmonizing the three components of internal power in Cloud Hands. Storing and projecting internal power, methods for training internal power, mental control over zhong ding, and the four major jin (Ward Off, Roll Back, Press, and Push) occupy the final three chapters.

This is a shortish book, but it's packed with important information. The target audience is the intermediate and advanced student rather than the beginner. This isn't to say that beginners can't gain something useful from it, but in my experience, beginners, who are still struggling to perform the form correctly, are not ready to appreciate some of the more refined aspects of Taiji. Not until, that is, they've settled into the basic movement patterns and can then turn their awareness to the inner workings of the body as it goes through the postures.

Tangora suggests that practitioners of other movement, healing, and martial arts also can benefit from what he has to say in this book. I think he's right, but I have to say that he is not as polished or conversational a writer as some of the other authors of excellent books on Taiji. But that doesn't mean he doesn't get his point across. He does, and the information is helpful as well as solid.

In addition, I really appreciate the way he focuses on one aspect of Taiji, and uses that to open up the entire art. Taiji is like that. The longer you practice, the more the intellectual aspects increase along with the physical and energetic. *The Internal Structure of Cloud Hands* exhibits depth, subtlety, and insight, and it does so in a way that few Taiji books have, to date. Perhaps Tangora has helped generate a new sort of Taiji book: the intense-focus type as opposed to the broad survey or thorough mapping. If so, I'm looking forward to more of this sort of thing from him—and from others.

PART II

The Taiji Classics

Biography of Wang Zhengnan
(Also known in abridged form as *Boxing Methods of the Internal School*)

By Huang Baijia
(Originally published 1676. *Brennan Translations*, 2014, 28 pages)

This is one of the oldest books reviewed in this series. The title is, *Biography of Wang Zhengnan*, but this short book is just as importantly about the codification of the internal school of martial arts.

The term *neijia* and the distinction between internal and external martial arts first appears in Huang Zongxi's 1669 *Epitaph for Wang Zhengnan*. Stanley Henning proposes that the *Epitaph*'s identification of the internal martial arts with the Taoism indigenous to China and of the external martial arts with the foreign Buddhism of Shaolin—and the Manchu Qing Dynasty to which Huang Zongxi was opposed—was an act of political defiance rather than one of technical classification. In 1676 Huang Zongxi's son, Huang Baijia, who learned martial arts from Wang Zhengnan, compiled the earliest extant manual of internal martial arts, the *Neijia quanfa*.[1]

The book under consideration is that very book. It begins with a short and sketchy history of the internal martial arts. From there, the author dips into an amusing section on the names Wang gave to his boxing art, none of which can be found in modern Taiji forms. Here are a few examples:

> Swinging an Elbow to Force the Door
> Caving in with Your Chest to Pound His Ribs
> Dark Clouds Hiding the Moon
> Lifting up a Gold Piece

He then mentions a few acupoint targets and warns against bad habits, such as being lazy or a drunk. Thirty-five hand techniques come next, followed by eighteen stepping techniques. These latter aren't directions of movement but rather types of steps, i.e., crushing step, grinding step, withdrawing step, and so forth. He writes:

> These elements are all used within the Six Lines and the Ten Sections of Brocade.

He lists all of the lines and sections, but I'm not going to because almost all of the names in them are couched in incomprehensibly poetic terms, but Huang does discuss each in some detail.

After that, he digresses for a few pages on the art of archery, and continues with some of his personal background

The book ends with a chapter that contains Huang Zongxi's 1669 *Epitaph for Wang Zhengnan*, here called *Memorial Inscription for Wang Zhengnan*, which further characterizes this important internal martial artist.

Notes
1 "Wudang Quan." *Wikipedia*, https://en.wikipedia.org/wiki/Wudang_quan

Wang Zongyue's Taiji Boxing Treatise
Appended with My Preface and "Five-Word Formula"

By Li Yiyu
(Handwritten manual, 1881. *Brennan Translations*, 2013, 30 pages)

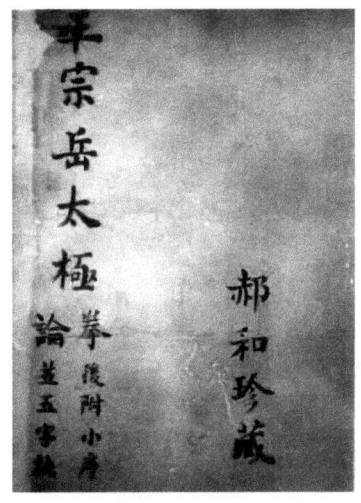

This book represents the earliest rendering of the "Salt Shop" Taiji Classic attributed to Wang Tsungyueh, a legendary Taiji exponent who supposedly helped disseminate Taiji prior to the Chen family's possession of the style. The book also has been attributed to Li Yiyu, himself, but scholars examining the very different writing styles of Li's other writings and of the Wang Classic appear to have laid that theory to rest.

Up first is the famous "Song of the Thirteen Dynamics," with the original text followed by Li's commentary on it. Li then ventures into Wang's essentials of playing hands (push hands) and understanding how to practice Taiji. This goes on for several chapters before ending at a "preface" by Li that dips a toe into the ocean of Taiji history.

The Five-Word Formula appears next:

1) The mind is calm.
2) The body is lively.
3) The energy is collected.
4) The power is complete.
5) The spirit is gathered.

Each has explanatory text. The final chapter is "The Trick to Releasing," which delves into how the previously stated Five-Word Formula provides clues to releasing fa jin energy. This ends the book.

I haven't relayed the details of each chapter of this book because I've gone into Wang's Classics elsewhere in this series. But that doesn't mean you shouldn't download and pick up this version. It is definitely an important seminal work on Taiji, and while it has been featured in perhaps hundreds of translations since it was discovered, this version, folks, is the real deal, straight from the Salt Shop to your door.

The Essence of T'ai Chi Ch'uan
The Literary Tradition

Translated and edited by Benjamin Pang Jeng Lo
   with Martin Inn, Robert Amacker, and Susan Foe
(North Atlantic Books, 1985, 100 pages)

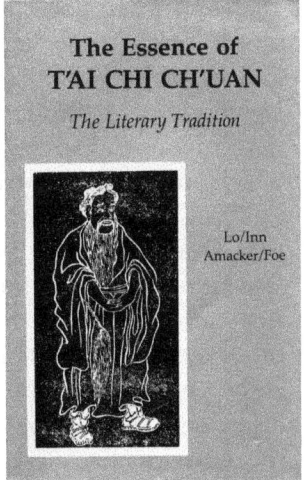

The Essence of T'ai Chi Ch'uan: The Literary Tradition, is a translation of the Taiji Classics, the seminal writings on the art dating from the early decades of the 20th century all the way back to the legendary founder of Taiji, Chang Sanfeng. As such, it, like most translations of the Classics, is incomplete. But I'm not sure I could name one single book that contains all the known classics under one cover, so that isn't really a criticism. The Classics in their entirety can have a fair amount of verbiage that isn't necessarily specific to the point of Taiji, so pulling the more meaningful statements from those that are less significant or overly cryptic, as the translators do here, is a perfectly valid editorial tool.

   The Essence of T'ai Chi Ch'uan presents a number of important Classics. Most are in poetic form, but that's not unusual for these writings, many of which originally were poems, often called "songs." In the case of this book, some of the statements in the Classics are broken out as individual poems presented on individual pages, rather than in their original extended forms. You could almost call this ta "short form" version of the Classics. But just as a short Taiji form still retains the essence of the art, so do these. And not all the Classics in these pages are short poems. There are a lot of more-extended prose pieces here, too.

I'm a huge fan of the Taiji Classics and read them often in one version or another. Some people note that they tend to affirm principles already learned rather than present specific instructional material. You read the statement but don't understand it until later, after you learn what it means. Then you read it again and say, "A-ha!" There may be some truth to that, and I've often experienced that. But the words can be instructive, too, introducing ideas that then find a home in one's form. For example, I read in the Classics about the sensation of "suspending the crown of the head as if by a string," or alternately, feeling a "light and sensitive energy at the top of the head," but in the beginning, those statements were just words. But they caused me to start trying to sense that suspension, and later, when I felt the sensation for myself, the recognition that it was an actual principle was important and helped lead me to loosening my waist and gaining a more flexible connection between my legs and torso. So, it could be said that the Classics don't teach movements but present the basic principles and tenets of Taiji, which are just as important in achieving correct practice.

When it comes to translations, this is a pretty good one and justly well known. If it's missing anything, it's expert commentary from the authors—or at least from Benjamin Lo, who was, at the time of first publication, the expert among the authors. There are several other excellent translations of the Classics in which the translator/author endeavors to further explain, from his or her own experiences and perspectives, what the sometimes cryptic statements of the Classics actually—or might—mean, and that's a helpful tool missing here. But sometimes, you just want to read the Classics without interference, interruption, or demands for specific ways of thinking, and the text of this version will deliver the goods.

T'ai-chi Touchstones
Yang Family Secret Transmissions

Compiled and translated by Douglas Wile
(Sweet Ch'i Press, 1983, 160 pages)

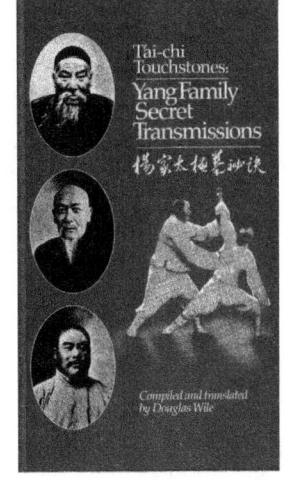

The foundational writings on Taiji, collectively called the Taiji Classics, are a group of eight or nine texts (depending on how one counts), each containing various numbers of "chapters" or "songs." These texts were accumulated from several locations in China during the 19th and early 20th centuries—primarily from a salt shop in Wuyang County, Henan; a manuscript discovered in a Beijing bookstall; and holdings by the Yang family. They are, so far, the earliest known writings on Taiji.

Tai Chi Touchstones: Yang Family Secret Transmissions, compiled and edited by Douglas Wile, is one of the more extensive and well-translated English-language versions of the original group of the Classics. Sweet Ch'i Press must be very glad that they published it, since not only is it a perennial seller, it is one of the more important books available in English on Taiji.

Wile is no slouch when it comes to Taiji history. For many years, he served as professor of Chinese language and literature at Brooklyn College. He is an expert translator as well as a scholar of Chinese history, in general, and is the author of several books on Taiji and other Chinese yogic practices. (See a review of his *Lost T'ai-chi Classics from the Late Ch'ing Dynasty*, below.) In this volume, he limits his personal commentary to a seven-page "Translator's Note," which lays out the difficulties in tracing Taiji's history—not just prior to the Chen family's acquisition of the art, but even into the 20th century. This brief chapter also delves into the history of the Classics and a few of the problems of dating and authorship attached to them.

The rest of this solid volume is devoted entirely to Wile's translation of the Classics. I've read a lot of versions of the Classics over the past forty-plus years, and many are excellent, but none are better or more complete than Wile's. His translation is very straightforward and does not attempt to further "poeticize" the texts, as some translations try to do. And each of the texts is attributed to its purported author, while many other translations or compilations of the Classics simply mush the texts together without attribution.

In addition, although a great many writers who include the Classics in their books also accompany them with commentaries that explain—with varying success—the sometimes obscure meaning contained in their often poetic and cryptic language, Wile eschews this, allowing the Classics to stand alone. I like many of the versions with commentaries a great deal. When it comes to learning more about Taiji, I'll take all the help I can get. But I also appreciate the fact that Wile lets the Classics speak for themselves. Jewels such as this need no setting.

As I said, I've read a great many versions of the Classics, but I never tire of them. When I first read them, they frequently came across as obscure, and I usually didn't know that they were talking about. The second time I read them, after I'd practiced Taiji for a little longer, I realized that I understood one or two elements. The third time, I understood more. And so it's gone. As my understanding of the art has grown, so has my comprehension of the Classics, which, as Wile's title implies, are not simply instructional notes but touchstones for advancement.

Thanks to Wile, it is possible to own a comprehensive and well-translated version of the original Taiji Classics under one cover. This is one of the few Taiji books that I've given as gifts, it's one I keep going back to, and it's one that should be in every Taiji library.

Lost T'ai-chi Classics from the Late Ch'ing Dynasty

by Douglas Wile
(State University of New York Press, 1996, 234 pages)

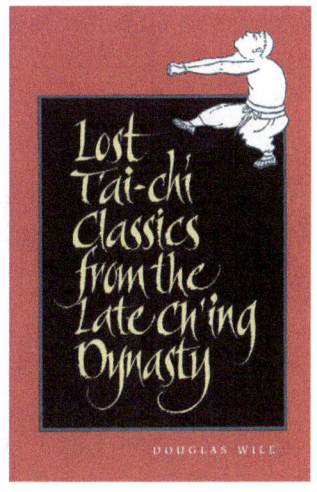

Douglas Wile follows his *T'ai-chi Touchstones: Yang Family Secret Transmissions* with yet another exegesis of the Taiji Classics titled *Lost T'ai Chi Classics from the Late Ch'ing Dynasty*. In the former volume (reviewed above), Wile, a professor of Chinese language and literature at Brooklyn College, limited his commentary on the texts of the Classics to introductory notes, leaving to the Classics the lion's share of the book to speak for themselves. In this book, he presents a newly released group of old writings on Taiji with his usual excellence of translation, but he also includes accompanying commentary that delves extensively into the history and purported authorship of these texts.

These are no small matters, and they have aroused the interest—and occasionally ire—of many Taiji factions. Just where did these texts come from? Was Chang Sanfeng really the author of three of them? And what about the historicity of Wang Tsungyeuh, who is the attributed author of several of the texts and who purportedly taught Taiji to the Chen family? These are just a few of the issues Wile deals with as he presents these newly discovered texts for the first time in English.

Only about half the book is occupied by the texts and Wile's commentaries. The second half contains numerous appendices. The first presents the texts in their original Chinese, and those that follow are primarily analyses of specific textual elements in an effort to determine the identity of the actual author and source material. As such, they will appeal primarily to historians of Taiji rather than to the general reader seeking information. But then, this is a scholarly work as much as it is a presentation of new material.

The new texts are, by and large, important additions to the Classics, and the book is valuable for that reason alone. More, Wile's commentaries not only delineate the content of the texts, but greatly expand our understanding of the milieu from with they rose. In particular, they affirm the critical importance of Wu Yuhsiang in the collection and dissemination of the Classics. (Note that this is the Wu who learned from the Chens and Yangs, whose style eventually became known as Wu/Hao Style. He is not related to the Wu family descended from Wu Quanyu, who founded Wu Family Style.)

Reading this book made me appreciate Wile's efforts all the more. I am an avid fan of the Classics, and, as with other important material on Taiji, the more the merrier. At the same time, the historical material made me hunger for a comprehensive and scholarly work on the development of Taiji. It would be a daunting task, but one I'd like to see Wile undertake.

As for this book: buy it, read it, and put it on the shelf next to *T'ai-chi Touchstones: Yang Family Secret Transmissions*. Later, read both again. You won't be sorry.

Taijiquan Theory of Dr. Yang, Jwing-Ming
The Root of Taijiquan

by Yang, Jwing-Ming
(YMAA Publication Center, 2003, 270 pages)

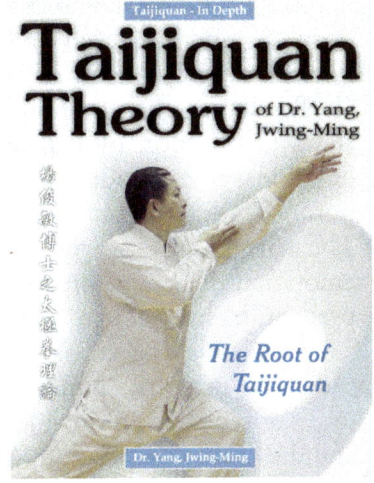

Yang Jwing-Ming is not only a proficient and significant martial artist of historical note, he also is an equally proficient and generous author who always seems sincere in his desire to impart what he knows to others. *Taijiquan Theory* is no exception. Its text is a compendium of songs and poems from the Taiji Classics, though the exact sources remain unnamed. Following the pattern of some of his other books —*Tai Chi Secrets of the Wu Style*, for example (see Volume VII of this series)—Yang presents each Classic in three forms: the original text in Chinese characters, a direct translation, and a more readable paraphrase of the translation, often with commentary.

The book is structured in ten parts, each one covering a particular aspect of Taiji. Following forwards by Grandmasters Li Maoching and Abraham Liu and a preface by the author, Yang begins the body text with a section on the general concepts of Taiji. In it, he explores the roots of the concept of Taiji in the *I Ching* and other ancient Chinese writings, and he includes some background on the taijitu—the tai chi symbol—and how it depicts movement. In this section, he also goes into the basics of chi flow in the human body, defining the various meridians, vessels, and acupuncture points along those paths that are especially important for the Taijiquanist. The theory of yin and yang receives some in-depth treatment also, as does the general theory of Taiji's Thirteen Postures and the three frame sizes (stance heights) adopted by practitioners.

Part two introduces the concept of regulating the body, which entails regulating the breath, the emotional mind, the chi, and the spirit. Yang begins this by explaining how to regulate the body via stationary postures then moving postures. Each of the next four parts delves more deeply into these four regulations.

First, the author goes into regulating the breathing, and he covers the basics of abdominal breathing, beginning with natural breathing, moving on to reverse breathing, and finishing with embryonic breathing. The reasons for adopting each of these forms of breathing and how each of them affect the practitioner are covered in some detail.

Regulating the emotional mind is the topic of part four. Yang starts this section by explaining the importance of regulating the emotional mind—not just for fighting, though it is critical for that purpose—but for improving the quality of one's outlook on life. The principal subject covered here is the mutual dependence of the emotional mind and breathing, and that leads to the idea of comprehending human nature through Taiji.

Regulating the chi is covered in part five, beginning with the theory of using the mind to lead the chi. From there, Yang segues into the secrets of both the Small Circulation (Microcosmic Orbit) and the Grand Circulation (Macrocosmic Orbit). He introduces two breathing exercises designed to enhance the practitioner's manifestation and circulation of chi: Yongquan breathing, or breathing from the Bubbling Wells in the soles of the feet, and Four Gates Breathing, which adds the hearts of the palms to the process. As if this isn't enough, there follows instruction on Five Gates Breathing, which adds the huiyin acupuncture point (located in the perineum). Taiji ball training finishes out the section.

Part six concerns regulating the spirit. This mostly entails raising the spirit energy to more highly activate the brain and opening the Third Eye. This requires the unification of spirit and chi.

Yang covers jin in the next part, beginning with a thesis of jin: what it is, how it is created, and how it is manifested. He explains the differences between external and internal jins, hard and soft jins, and long and short jins. The secret of jin, he maintains, is in the way one coordinates breathing with the expression of a movement. Last, he talks about storing jin and practicing the "heng" and "ha" sounds to enhance the power and expression of jin.

Pushing hands is covered in part eight. First, Yang describes the basics of push hands and its theory, then he proceeds to detail several push hands forms and practice methods. He also discusses rooting, and he gives a number of practical exercises to establish a root and strengthen and deepen it over time. Practicing methods for the abilities of listening, following, attaching, and adhering come next, and then Yang goes into the six turning secrets of Taiji: circling, spinning, rotating, twisting, coiling, and spiraling.

Sparring is the subject of the next part, and here the author goes into various aspects of kicking, striking, wrestling, and chin na. Included are the concepts of the "central door" and "empty door," both of which are tactical ways to approach an opponent, and the concepts of the "sky window" and the "ground wicket," both of which are natural openings in an opponent's defenses. Several paired fighting strategies are covered in some detail—long and short, hard and soft, advancing and retreating—and these are embellished by a discussion of timing and what Yang calls the "Theory of the Fight of No Fight."

Part ten concludes the principal text, and here the work ventures into the philosophical. The book finishes with a glossary and an index.

The text is enlivened by a number of photos, illustration, charts, and diagrams, some of which seem a bit arcane, though most are helpful in furthering the reader's understanding. If I have a criticism, it's that the title is misleading since the theories presented are taken from the Taiji Classics. Perhaps it ought to be titled, *Taijiquan Theory Compiled and Translated by Dr. Yang, Jwing-Ming*. And I do wish the author had cited the sources of the original writings.

Those concerns aside, I have to say that Yang's commentaries are one of the most complete and thorough analyses of the texts I've ever read. All-in-all, this is another excellent offering from a master of the Chinese martial arts and of writing about them, and it is well worth adding to one's martial arts library.

Tai Chi Chuan
Decoding the Classics for the Modern Martial Artist

By Dan Docherty
(The Crowood Press, 2009, 142 pages)

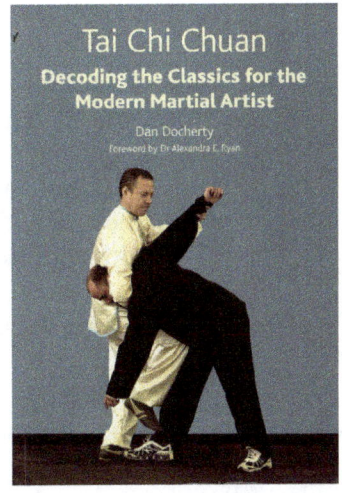

Tai Chi Chuan: Decoding the Classics for the Modern Martial Artist, by Dan Docherty, is not a book to be taken lightly. And I do not intend to despite the fact that it stirred up such negative impressions while I read it that I found myself wanting to punt on reviewing it. But here it is, here I am, and reviewing the the bad and the ugly as well as the good is part of the job. As for this book, it's schizophrenic in the sense that it is both very good and very bad at the same time. And it's certainly ugly, too.

The author is a Wudang Taiji stylist. Here's a tidbit on him from the *Wikipedia* article on Wudang Taiji:

> Dan Docherty was born in Glasgow, Scotland, in 1954. He graduated with an LLB in 1974 and soon after moved to Hong Kong where he served as an inspector in the Royal Hong Kong Police Force until 1984. Soon after he arrived in Hong Kong in 1975 he started training t'ai chi ch'uan under Cheng Tinhung and within a few years was elected to represent Hong Kong in full-contact fighting competitions. In 1980 he won the Open Weight Division at the 5th South East Asian Chinese Pugilistic Championships in Malaysia. In 1985

he was awarded a Postgraduate Diploma in Chinese from Ealing College, London. He is now based in London and travels extensively teaching and writing about t'ai chi ch'uan.[1]

I think it's safe to say that Docherty really has the chops to write in-depth on Taiji, and as long as he sticks to technical matters, his information is most often excellent. But jeeze, his attitude is the pits. *Tai Chi Chuan: Decoding the Classics for the Modern Martial Artist* is a relatively slender book packed with good material, but it's also liberally salted with a bunch of opinionated and offensive BS. This seems to agree with this further information from the *Wikipedia* article:

> Mr. Docherty is known for his strong views on the history of t'ai chi ch'uan and is seen as a polarizing figure within the world of t'ai chi. In articles and interviews he has spoken of confrontations with other t'ai chi teachers, including an infamous meeting with one Shen Hong-xun, a master who claimed to have and to teach "empty force", or the ability to move a person without physical contact. The meeting ended up with Mr. Docherty pouring water over the head of Shen Hong-Xun, not to prove that empty force does not exist but to suggest that Master Shen was unable to summon and use it at that time.

Well, after reading this book, it's obvious that Docherty is as polarizing on the printed page as he must be in person. But let's complete our survey of the book before we go into specifics.

The general purpose of the book is to provide an in-depth exegesis of the Taiji Classics, those venerable writings on Taiji that serve as the art's founding documents. I'm not going to go into the basic history of the revelation of the Classics. That can be found, in one version or another, in a great number of Taiji books and manuals. But as with all Chinese martial arts manuals of the pre-Republican period, their true genesis and authorship are frequently called into question. Be that as it may, they remain vitally important to Taiji in laying out many of the principles and methodologies of the art. So, I generally welcome any addition that can be made in explicating these works for modern readers.

However....

The forward by Dr. Alexandra E. Ryan states:

> To my knowledge this is the first book in English to bring these materials together and with fresh translations as well as practical commentaries.

The author makes the same claim in his "Acknowledgements":

> This book presents the first fully illustrated translation and commentary on the Taiji Classics.... There are translations on the market already, but they are largely unsatisfactory, being written mainly by people who have little or no practical experience, and limited technical knowledge.

I don't know who Dr. Ryan is, but she and Docherty should have done a little research before they made these claims. This book was published in 2009, so let's see what earlier translations-plus-commentary were out there at the time. I can't do an absolutely thorough survey since I do not own all Taiji books in English printed prior to 2009, but I did quickly go through my library and easily found excellent earlier translations of the Classics, most with explanations and many with illustrations, in the following books, all of which are by acknowledged masters, not, as Docherty states, "by people who have little or no practical experience, and limited technical knowledge." Most obvious is *Taijiquan Theory* by Yang Jwing-ming, just reviewed, but others are:

Advanced Yang Style Tai Chi Chuan, Vol. One, by Yang Jwing-ming, 1986
Advanced Yang Style Tai Chi Chuan, Vol. Two by Yang Jwing-ming, 1986
Tai Chi Secrets of the Wu Style, by Yang Jwing-ming, 2002
Tai Chi Classics, Vol. 2, by Waysun Liao, 1977
Fundamentals of Tai Chi Ch'uan, by Wen-Shan Huang, 1979
The Tao of Tai-Chi Chuan, by Jou Tsung-hwa, 1980
Tai Chi Touchstones: Yang Family Secret Transmissions, by Douglas Wile, 1983
Lost Tai-chi Classics from the late Ch'ing Dynasty, by Douglas Wile, 1996

I hardly think that these authors, at least the first four named, are Taiji slackers. Nor are these the only versions of the Classics in my library—there are dozens more renditions, all reviewed in this series, many excellent and with expert commentary. And I'm sure others existed on the market prior to 2009 that I don't know about. But that doesn't mean we shouldn't have one more. Each rendition has the potential to add value to the reader's understanding and practice, thanks to the input of each individual author's perspective. And Docherty is up to delivering, at least on a professional level, being expert in both Taiji and Chinese language.

He begins with a section on the background of the Chinese martial arts, and it's easy to see why his take on kung fu history—and particularly Taiji history—is often considered controversial. As often occurs with practitioners of kung fu styles, he favors the importance of his own style in the genesis of his martial arts lineage—in this case, Wudang Taiji. However, his history is fairly thorough even if it does, like all such histories, rely too much on legend and supposition that skews in favor of his particular style. However, while he favors his own take on Taiji history, he does give a fair accounting of several alternative historical scenarios, some of which he derides, but some of which he credits with potential veracity.

Being versed in Chinese allows him to describe the various and often multifold meanings attached to certain Chinese words and terms. He goes into the difficulties of exactly translating Chinese to English—and even says the reverse also is true. This sort of disclaimer is enunciated by just about every translator of any language into any other language, and is such a truism that it really does not need mentioning. Docherty not only presents the various alternate meanings, he describes how they work together in a word or term to give it both poetic meaning and psychological depth. And he also explains why he chooses alternative translations of words and terms that often are at odds with choices commonly used by other translators.

Unfortunately, his reasoning doesn't always seems inevitably valid, and often, his personal choices seem to be pedantic, pointless, or even counterproductive. More on that later. For now, let's return to the survey.

As with many other translators, Docherty delivers a rendition in full of each of the five main Classics. Each rendition is followed by his explanations and clarifications. He begins with a couple of pieces of advice:

> Nowadays, many TCC students follow and attempt to copy the teacher's movements, and there is usually little explanation. Such students get something out of a study of the Classics, but the more limited their exposure to the varied elements in TCC, the more limited will be their ability to comprehend the Classics and to understand what they are doing.

This is weak criticism because this isn't really a "modern" issue. Students of traditional martial arts in China followed and attempted to copy the teacher's movements, often without explanation. So says the literature from the time and most historical accounts, virtually across styles from the hard to the soft, from north to south. It is reputed, for example, that when Yang Panhao took on Wu Quanyu as a student, he made Wu hold the single posture Stork Stands on One Leg every day for hours over a lengthy period of time, completely without explanation, before he taught him anything else.

Docherty continues:

> The TCC Classics are aimed at those who are at a level beyond that of the beginner or dilettante. The vast majority of practitioners don't have the knowledge to interpret and follow the fascinating and insightful material in the TCC Classics, which can, like philosophical classics, be of use to anyone who has the resolve to apply them. Incorrect understanding leads to incorrect practice.

This might be true in some sort of absolutist sense, but according to Docherty, we must eschew the Classics when we are beginners, because only the experienced (such as him) are able to get anything out of these writings. This seems patently arrogant and ignores the methodology of learning, in which curiosity feeds examination, which in turn feeds development that then leads to more curiosity. Docherty even gives lie to his own disbelief that beginners and dilettantes can get anything out of the Taiji Classics in the latter part of the sentence: "the TCC Classics, which can, like philosophical classics, be of use to anyone who has the resolve to apply them." Can't beginners or dilettantes have such a resolve to apply them, as well, if not as deeply, as more seasoned practitioners? I believe they can.

My own experience with the Classics began soon after I began learning Taiji, and, yes, I didn't understand much of anything in them at the time. But I absorbed some of the hints and clues, and a year later, I read them again and understood a couple of things that my practice had taught me. These were elements I didn't know I'd learned until the Classics revealed something about them. At the same time, I noticed additional statements that sparked my curiosity and subsequently led me to explore the concepts they discussed, leading to later revelations in my practice. And the more I read the Classics over the following decades, the more of them I comprehended and the more clues appeared to further my practice. This back-and-forth began with my initial state of total ignorance and continues to this day with my perpetual state of total ignorance.

But for Docherty, I now comprehend some measure of the Classics only because I now have experience that I didn't have before. Yet I've always gotten something from reading them and letting them lead me to observe and experiment, guiding me even in my ignorance. So, some understanding the Classics does come with experience over time, as Docherty says, but one does not have to fully understand them to benefit and gain clues from reading them.

Docherty states that the five Classics he translates in this book are the most significant—and perhaps only "real"—Classics, though in point of fact, many more Classics exist in the complete canon, most from the pre-Republican period, a number of which have been translated by others, notably Douglas Wile.[2] But it is true, as Docherty states, that these five are the most significant. The Classics Docherty translates and explicates are (using his titles):

1) *The Taiji Chuan Discourse (Taiji Chuan Lun)*
   Also titled: *Taiji Chuan Treatise*
   Attributed to Chang San-feng

2) *The Canon of Taiji Chuan (Taiji Chuan Ching)*
   Also titled: *Theory of Taiji Chuan and Taiji Chuan Classic*
   Attributed to Wang Zong-yue (Wang Tsung-yueh)

3) *Interpretation of the Practice of the Thirteen Tactics* (*Shi San Shi Xing Gong Xin Jie*)
(Also titled: *Treatise on the Practice of the Thirteen Movements/ Postures/Methods*; *Thirteen Postures: Comprehending External and Internal Training*; and *Mental Elucidation of the Practice of Taiji Chuan*)
Usually attributed to Yang Lu-chan's student, Wu Yuxiang (Wu Yuhsiang)

4) *Song of the Thirteen Tactics* (*Shi San Shi Ge*)
(Also titled: *Song of the Thirteen Movements/Postures/Methods*)
Author unknown

5) *The Fighter's Song* (*Da Shou Ge*)
(Also titled: *Song of Pushing Hands* and *Song of Sparring*)
Author unknown

At the outset, the author spends some energy discussing the differences between literal and "artistic" translation, coming down strongly on the side of the literalists, though at the same time complaining about the impossibility of accurate literal translation. That disclaimer notwithstanding, by and large, his translations are readable and informative in their own right, and his explications generally focus the reader on the several important points of each passage with convincing arguments and examples. But not always.

Unfortunately, Docherty's expertise is seriously marred by his blatant desire to be the No. 1 authority on Taiji—and it seems, everything else. According to Docherty, there is one major problem with all other translations of the Classics. They weren't translated by that paragon of Taiji understanding and Chinese-to-English translation: Dan Docherty. The simple truth for Docherty is that no one knows much of anything worth knowing about Taiji except Dan Docherty. It's his way or the highway. So, since Docherty lauds his own translation above others, let's look at it. I'm not going to attempt a side-by-side comparison of his work with the work of other translators of the Classics. That would take a whole book, and who the heck would actually read it? But we can look at the author's modus and method.

While Docherty usually does the reader a service by giving alternative meanings to common Taiji terms and concepts, he often is harshly adamant about his personal choices. And he often lapses into the pedantic through his resolute use of Chinese terms where translated English terms would better serve the English-reading audience. For example, he always employs the terms Peng, Lu, Ji, and An instead of the English versions: Wardoff Rollback, Press, and Push. Okay, maybe those are the "correct" terms—at least in Chinese—but the readers of this book live mostly in the English-speaking world. I don't need to dress in Chinese clothing to practice Taiji.

And in the inverse, he persistently uses alternative translations of common Taiji terms and concepts to no real effect or apparent point other than to prove his erudition. He's probably just as correct in most instances as are other translations, and usually his translations add to the reader's understanding, such as his version of the title to Classic five. Usually translated as, "Song of Pushing Hands," it is rendered by Docherty as "The Fighter's Song." His rationale is that, while this Classic makes no mention of push hands, it does discuss aspects of fighting.

Okay, I can go along with that, but then he turns around and says:

> Xin Jie is "interpretation"/"explanation," something many Chinese concepts require before they can be understood. I've translated "Shi San Shi" as Thirteen Tactics rather than Thirteen Movements/Postures, because every technique in the form is supposed to be derived from a combination of one of the Five Steps and the Eight Forces, so their possible permutations are much more varied that would appear from the latter translation.

Pardon me, but the first word in the term resolutely remains "thirteen." Thirteen this, thirteen that. It doesn't matter what or which, it's still thirteen, and thirteen does not literally mean "all permutations" no matter what anyone says. It means thirteen. And the idea of the Thirteen Whatevers combining into and spawning "all permutations" holds true no matter what you choose for the second word, whether you prefer "tactics," "postures," "dynamics," or "movements." You could call them "Thirteen Pollywogs" as long as you adhere to Taiji's correct thirteen parameters. Anyway, tactics aren't techniques. Tactics are abstract concepts, not physical manifestations, and these Thirteen Whatevers are all physical and physiological manifestations. More properly, they really are "movements," and only appear to be "postures" in static photos of the form, though they often are defined by the terminal postures in which where the energy of a movement terminates.

Another example is Docherty's gripe with the use of the term jin.

> Many Chinese characters have been wrongly or poorly translated. "Jin" is usually translated as "energy," when it means "trained force."

Well, no. Most translations of jin that I've come across make a definite effort to refer to jin as a "trained force" that imparts "energy," not as the sort of vague, namby-pamby concept as implied by Docherty. And most writers on Taiji almost always go to extra lengths to distinguish jin from li (strength) or from force that has neither focus nor intent.

I do have to laud the author, however, for providing a translation of General Qi Ji-Guang's *Classic of Boxing*, which appears following the explanations of the five major Classics. At the outset of it, he admits that he's not going into as much detail as he has with the five major Classics. True. He does go into every point, but his explication of this work is not the thorough exegesis that he largely delivered elsewhere. Despite the lite commentary, this chapter probably is the most valuable one in the book, primarily because this particular Classic is rare in English-language Taiji literature. So kudos to Docherty for presenting it.

However, his translation of it can be pretty darn obscure or confusing as well as cursory, calling into question the wisdom of literal translation over the more artistic sort, especially when Docherty embeds fragments of commentary within the passage. Take this, for example:

> Though Lu Hong's Eight Movements are hard, and do not attain the level of Cotton Zhang's (cotton (mian) – here, as in the TCC Classics, it means soft) Short Striking (close quarter fighting), the legs of Li bantian from Shandong (bantian is probably a nickname: half heaven – half of

Shandong province had heard of him); Eagle Claw Wang's holds (a reference to Qinna – seizing and holding), the throws of Thousand Falls Zhang, Zhang Bo-jing's striking, the staff method of the Shaolin Temple, and the Qingtian staff method simultaneously (Qingtian is a famous place for boxing); the Yang family spear method and Bazi Boxing and staff, all are now famous.

Tell the truth, now. Did you have to read that more than once to get the meaning? I mean, jeeze, that's *one* sentence! If you ignore all the subordinate clauses of this convoluted piece of work, you can understand what Docherty is saying. But you, dear reader, shouldn't have to do that. As the writer, Docherty's job was to provide not just an accurate translation, but a readable one. But his insistence on literality, even when literality is the enemy, causes him to drop the ball not just here, but elsewhere. Such as this gem:

All breathing is done through the nose, so the air is filtered by the mucous membranes and warmed before it goes into the lungs. By developing relaxation through slow practice of form and Taiji Nei Kung, the lungs are able to expand further down than normal. This process can be seen and felt a the area of the Dan Tian. Ironically, this is bad new for smokers, because they are able to inhale more effectively.

Okay, I get the part about deep abdominal breathing being not only healthful but essential to Taiji. Sure. But I'm not sure about deep breathing being bad news for smokers. I suppose he means that if smokers learn to breathe more deeply, they'll inhale cigarette smoke more deeply, causing deeper damage. But really, are smokers likely to be practicing deep-breathing chi kung? Those who do, probably quit smoking soon after. And darn, I never knew that smoking actually causes one to inhale more effectively. Maybe that's because it isn't so. I smoked as a youth, and as soon as I *quit*, I could inhale more effectively.

The long and short of it is that when a translator insists that all other translations are either incorrect, lacking, or faulty except for his own, and his own are often contrary to the majority and pretty faulty themselves, then that translator's work is equally suspect by the translator's own rules. And Docherty often slides into territory that is suspect or faulty. The truth is, people do what they want to do (what their spirit instructs, if they're lucky), and it is ethically disingenuous to deny them their methods unless you want them to deny you yours. Nobody in this world is right all the time, though some seem to be perpetually in the wrong.

In addition to Docherty's translation faux pas, I also found other elements of this book annoying or downright distasteful. For example, Docherty often mentions some fact or facet only to ignore any explanation. When discussing Bend the Bow, Shoot the Tiger, for instance, he says this:

> The body is bent in order to straighten; when the bow is bent, there is tension, and when released, power goes to upper and lower extremities and arms and legs. Tiger is the opponent. Draw/bend the bow to shoot the Tiger is a classical TCC technique based on a Zen story.

Okay, but where's the story? If you're going to mention a story, then relate it. This book isn't all that long that it couldn't stand a little human padding. Otherwise, this sentence is meaningless except to give the author the opportunity to show his erudition and the reader's ignorance.

And sometimes he descends into reliance on "ancestors" to prove his point, such as his take on this statement from Classic Four: "Freely contract and extend, open and close and listen." Of this sentence, Docherty says:

> The second sentence paraphrases Lao Tzu's "To shrink something, you must first stretch it. To weaken something, you must first strengthen it. To take from something, you must first give to it." (p. 96–97)

The truth is, grandpa isn't always right. Lao Tzu's statement might be a universal truism, but it's not universally true. I can expand H_2O either by heating or freezing it. No shrinkage necessary—or even possible since water cannot be compressed by normal means. I can weaken iron by melting it. No prior strengthening needed. I can stretch a rubber band, but I can't really shrink it. All I can do is allow it to unstretch, which is not the same as shrinking. And greedy people regularly take from others but never give back. Docherty might be quoting Lao Tzu, but this statement is bull, even if I understand his basic meaning in terms of Taiji to be that one must initiate movement in one direction or particular way in order to execute a movement in a different direction or way. Taiji operates in a state in which yin and yang are distinguished, but reality, though replete with these two forces, is such a mixture that all sorts of non-yin/yang things happen within the parameters of local circumstance. The wind blows and ruffles my hair, but it never un-blows and brushes my hair down.

Docherty promises many photos and illustrations to aid in his explanations, and okay, he did include many photos and illustrations, but almost all of the photos are standard shots of applications. They might be intended to illustrate points in the text, but too often the explanations are lacking or are incomplete or vague, and the photos offer little inspiration. The only illustrations that are really germane are those included with General Qi Ji-Guang's *Classic of Boxing*, and these only historically because they are original to the text, not because they further understanding.

But all this isn't to say that there aren't smooth facets to this book as well as rough spots. I've already mentioned a few, and as I've said, the author is obviously expert and knowledgable. Most of the information he delivers is sound, interesting, and applicable to one's personal practice, no matter what the style. And when the author slams the wholesale commercialization of modern Taiji, I have to agree fully.

> Now we have Tai Chi (the Chuan or boxing has disappeared!) for golf, for skiing, for tennis. There is Aqua Tai Chi, Nudist Tai Chi, Tai Chi for diabetes and many more. Normal TCC practice can do all the things that people running these programmes claim to do, as well as a lot more that, because of their "fast food" approach, they fail to deliver. All this is really led by marketing, and those running the programmes are often better at commerce than at actual practice.

Likewise interesting is the story of Yang Chengfu's death. We often read about the lives of martial arts masters, but rarely about how they died. For anyone who wants to know why such a renowned master of an art that is supposed to confer longevity died at the relatively young age of fifty-three, Docherty has the goods. But it's his story, so I'll let him tell it.

Unfortunately, positive notes like these don't let Docherty off the hook when he too often extends pointless ad hominem attacks in the manner of online trolls and aims them at everyone not Docherty. His sweeping and overblown criticisms of not just other translators but of most Taiji practitioners border on the slanderous—or even the crank—with little foundation in anything but the author's own harsh attitudes that seem rooted in something other than Taiji expertise. So my real criticism of this book, beyond its pedantic nature and several weaknesses in translation, is of the author's distasteful melange of arrogance and unnecessary cruelty. Take this gem:

> There is now a plethora of oral instruction available on the internet either from pimple-faced teenage scribblers who can't find a girlfriend or burnt-out old soaks entering the second half of a wasted life.

His point is to find a qualified instructor to personally teach you, but this statement is entirely laughable as well as egregiously offensive. And patently incorrect. There might be a fair share of pimple-faced teenage scribblers and burnt-out old soaks (that must be me!) online, but there also are a very large number of acknowledged experts and masters, and it's pretty easy to tell the difference. Besides, that burnt-out old soak might not have lived a wasted life and might just have something valuable to offer. But of course, none of them count against Docherty's knowledge and skill.

Here's another example:

> It is polarity rather than duality that we are more likely to encounter when dealing the the cultural and the martial. This is immediately obvious when we read the books of academic writers on TCC They obviously have limited knowledge of the martial, but feel compelled to write about it; like eunuchs writing on the pleasures of love-making.

So, according to Docherty, everybody-not-Doherty who is writing about Taiji is either a pimple-faced teenager without a girlfriend, a burnt-out old soak, or an impotent academic who is totally ignorant of Taiji but writes about it anyway. And none of them have any skill to speak of. Jeeze. Like I said, it's all about Docherty.

I'm of the opinion that instructional texts should actually instruct, not obfuscate and confuse, and I'm afraid that this book does a bit of both. I can't fault Docherty for the real information in this book. It's all pretty solid as long as you remember that this is his take on matters, which is not necessarily better or worse than the interpretations of other expert authors on the subjects of Taiji, the Classics, and the art of translation—no matter what Docherty might think.

Regarding the history of Taiji, he, like many others, favors his own style's place in the systematic development of the art, whether it deserves that position or not. Who's to say, really? Taiji's history is so rooted in legend, surmise, wishful thinking, and even deliberate obfuscation that any somewhat learned discussion of the matter is bound to mix fiction and guesswork with the facts.

Unfortunately, Docherty often seems more intent on displaying his expertise in Taiji and his erudition regarding Chinese texts while neglecting the stated purpose of this book, which is to present a faithful rendition and expert explication of the Taijiquan Classics. The space he wastes with his opinionated slurs of others could have been used more productively to actually say something worth saying.

Notes

1 "Wudang T'ai Chi Ch'uan." *Wikipedia*, https://en.wikipedia.org/wiki/Wudang_t'ai_chi_ch'uan
2 "Tai Chi Classics." *Wikipedia*, https://en.wikipedia.org/wiki/T%27ai_chi_classics

Phosphene Publishing Company
publishes books and DVDs relating to literature,
history, the paranormal, film, spirituality, and the
martial arts.

For other great titles, visit
phosphenepublishing.com

www.ingramcontent.com/pod-product-compliance
Lightning Source LLC
Chambersburg PA
CBHW050109170426
43198CB00014B/2510